# THE FAT LOSS
# HANDBOOK

**Other books by these authors**

Egger, G. and Stanton, R.; *The GutBuster 'Waist Loss' Guide for men*

Egger, G. and Stanton, R., *GutBuster 2: The High Energy Guide*

Egger, G. and Champion, N., *The Fitness Leader's Handbook*

Egger, G., Champion, N. and Hurst, G., *The Fitness Leader's Exercise Bible*

Egger, G., Spark, R. and Lawson, J., *Health Promotion Strategies and Methods*

Egger, G., Spark, R. and Donovan, R., *Health and the Media*

Egger, G. *The Sport Drug*

# The fat loss handbook

## A guide for professionals

Dr Garry Egger
and
Dr Boyd Swinburn

ALLEN & UNWIN

This edition published in 1996 by
Allen & Unwin
9 Atchison Street, St Leonards NSW 2065 Australia
Phone: (61 2) 9901 4088
Fax:    (61 2) 9906 2218
E-mail: 100252.103@compuserve.com

National Library of Australia
Cataloguing-in-Publication entry:

Egger, Garry.
   The fat loss handbook: a guide for professionals.

   Includes index.
   ISBN 1 86448 135 8.

   1. Weight loss. 2. Obesity. 3. Reducing diets.
   I. Swinburn, Boyd A. II. Title

616.39806

Set in 10.5/12 pt Garamond by DOCUPRO, Sydney
Printed by Australian Print Group

10 9 8 7 6 5 4 3 2 1

# Contents

# Figures

# Tables

# Contributors

*Authors*

**Garry Egger MPH PhD** Director, Centre for Health Promotion and Research, Sydney; Clinical Lecturer, Centre for Health Advancement, School of Medicine, University of Newcastle; Scientific Director, 'GutBusters' Pty Ltd, Sydney.
**Boyd Swinburn MD, MBChB, FRACP** Medical Director, National Heart Foundation of New Zealand; Senior Research Fellow, Department of Community Health, School of Medicine, Auckland.

*Other contributing authors*

**Alan Bolton BHMS (Hons)** Fitness Consultant; Sydney.
Chapter 4: Bioenergetics and energy metabolism; Chapter 12: Movement and fat loss; Chapter 13: Individualised movement prescription for fat loss
**Matthew Fischer BSc(Hons) PhD** Dietitian, Victorian Department of Health, Melbourne.
Chapter 11: 'Fad diets' and dieting for fat loss
**Matthew O'Neill BBSpSc, MSc (Nutrition and Dietetics)** Dietitian, Sydney.
Chapter 8: Dietary fat and how to reduce it; Chapter 9: Dietary carbohydrate and how to increase it; Chapter 10: Hunger and appetite
**James Ritchie MB, BS, FRCS(ENG), FRACS** General surgeon, Sydney.
Chapter 19: Drugs and surgical treatment
**Grant Taylor MSc(Hons), DipClinPsych, MNZPS, MNZCCPsych**

Clinical and health psychologist, Auckland.
Chapter 21: Ethical issues in obesity treatment
**Hilary Tupling BA(Hons) Psychology** Clinical Psychologist, Sydney.
Chapter 17: Behavioural influences; Chapter 20: Eating disorders

# Abbreviations

| | |
|---|---|
| ADI | abdominal diameter index |
| ADP | adenosine diphosphate |
| ATP | adenosine triphosphate |
| BIA | bio-impedance analysis |
| BMI | body mass index |
| BW | body weight |
| CR | conditioned response |
| CrP | creatine phosphate |
| CS | conditioned stimulus |
| CT | computerised tomography |
| DEXA | dual energy X-ray absorptiometry |
| EE | energy expenditure |
| EI | energy intake |
| EPOC | excess post-exercise oxygen consumption |
| FFA | free fatty acids |
| FFM | fat-free mass |
| FITT | frequency, intensity, time and type |
| FM | fat mass |
| FT | fast twitch muscle fibre |
| GI | glycaemic index |
| GIT | gastrointestinal tract |
| HRT | hormone replacement therapy |
| LBM | lean body mass |
| LPL | lipoprotein lipose |
| MR | metabolic rate |
| MRI | magnetic resonance imaging |
| MSG | monosodium glutamate |
| MUFA | monounsaturated fatty acid |

NIDDM  non insulin dependent diabetes mellitus
NIR    near infrared analysis
OSA    obstructive sleep apnoea
PUFA   polyunsaturated fatty acid
RET    rational emotive therapy
RMR    resting metabolic rate
RQ     respiratory quotient
RT     resistance training
SAD    sagittal diameter
SCFA   short chain fatty acid
SE     socio-economic
SFQ    short fat questionnaire
SI     satiety index
SPA    spontaneous physical activity
ST     slow twitch muscle fibre
TEF    thermic effect of food
TGs    triglycerides
UR     unconditioned response
US     unconditioned stimulus
VMN    ventromedial hypothalamus
WHR    waist-to-hip ratio

# Introduction
# The need for a handbook on fat loss

Why a handbook for 'fat loss leaders', or those working in the weight control industry? That's a question that could have been asked back in the early 1980s when the new-style fitness industry took over the care of the modern body. One of the major goals of the fitness industry was then, and still is, decreasing body fatness. But the fitness industry went a little off track. Its emphasis on competitive aerobics and the body beautiful tended to overlook that large section of the population that actually has a problem with fatness, but doesn't necessarily want to achieve high level fitness or the 'ideal physique'.

The so-called exercise 'boom' did have a big impact on research into muscle physiology and exercise science. It's probably not exaggerating to say that more was learned in the decade of the 1980s about muscle function, than in the whole of human history before this. Yet search the academic shelves for *scientifically factual* practical advice on fat loss, and you'll find them bare. There are, of course, the myriad of weight control books and programs promising magical outcomes for minuscule effort. But there is little with an adequate research base that is understandable at the lay level, for people who potentially might help others in this area.

This book provides practical information based on a new model of weight control, developed as a result of the failure of previous paradigms to explain the growth of overfatness and obesity in the community. It is not meant to turn someone into a dietitian or an exercise scientist. It is meant to complement these practices by providing practical advice that can be used by those interested or involved in fat loss. The first part of the book

(Chapters 1–6) provides background and a rationale for the information to follow. The model is spelled out in Chapter 7 and the remainder of the book is then taken up with expounding sections of the proposed model.

In developing this approach, we are conscious of the need to not stigmatise those very obese people who have a genuine genetic base to their obesity, for whom the maintenance of a low level of body fat is difficult and the attainment of a 'model-type' figure is impossible. Our main concern is with the growth of obesity in the general community and the potential long-term health effects of this, both at the individual and the public health level.

Obesity and overfatness in this sense should not be seen as an aesthetic issue, but one of health and quality of life. Knowledge of causes, potential treatments and, perhaps more importantly, prevention in future generations, is vital for the future. We hope we have contributed to this knowledge.

Garry Egger and Boyd Swinburn, 1996

# I
# DEALING WITH OVERFATNESS AND OBESITY

# 1
# Overfatness and obesity into the 21st century

### SUMMARY OF MAIN POINTS

- Almost 1 in 2 people in western countries are now defined as overweight or obese.
- People in some Western countries have been increasing body weight at the average rate of 1g/day over the last decade.
- 'Overfatness' is a more appropriate term than 'overweight'.
- The fitness and nutrition booms have had little impact on levels of fatness throughout the world.
- The environment determines prevalence, and genes determine the presence of obesity.
- The traditional paradigm of 'weight=energy in (food)—energy out (exercise) is no longer adequate for understanding obesity.

In recent times there has been regular mention made of a 'fitness boom' in Western societies. Gyms, it was thought, were bursting at the seams; streets were littered with runners and recreation facilities were overflowing. Similarly, there has been a nutrition boom with people becoming more aware of healthy eating patterns and reducing their fat intake. As a result, Western populations should be increasingly leaner and fitter. The reality, however, is different. By the mid 1990s it became clear that the developed world was facing an epidemic of obesity.[1] Figures as high as 1 in 2 people in countries such as the US, Russia, the UK, Australia and New Zealand are overfat or obese and the proportion is rising at an increasing rate.[2]

In Australia, Dr Stan Bennett from the Australian Institute of Health, has estimated that the average Australian has been putting on weight at the rate of 1g/day over the past decade (around 3kg every 10 years). Even amongst teenagers the proportion who are overweight has risen to around one-third of all 12–20 year olds. Despite the huge expenditure on weight control products and services (estimated to be around $10 billion per annum in the US)[3], people are getting fatter. How could this happen? One of the major concerns of the fitness industry in the past has been decreasing body fatness, but the industry went a little off the track. Its emphasis on competitive aerobics and the body beautiful tended to overlook that large section of the population that actually has a problem with fatness, but doesn't necessarily want to achieve high level fitness.

In the early 1980s approximately 15 per cent of the North American and Australian populations were exercising at a level that was considered, then, to provide cardiovascular fitness. It has been estimated that only 1–2 per cent of the population regularly use an organised gym or fitness centre to do this. It's quite obvious from looking inside a gym that most of the people who attend are already lean and fit and are just trying to get *leaner* and *fitter*. As time has progressed, these figures have changed little. So although we've been through what is often called a 'fitness boom', the concentration of effort amongst those who are already active, tends to make this more of a fitness 'pop'!

## FATNESS AND FITNESS

There are still large sections of Western populations who are classified as totally sedentary or inactive, i.e. they don't do any regular physical activity in their leisure time (see Table 1.1). It's quite likely that a large proportion of these people also make up that section of the population regarded as overweight or obese (see Table 1.2). They are unlikely to spring from their lounge chairs into an aerobics class, even though they may wish to decrease their own creeping corpulence. To them, fitness is anathema. They'd like to be less fat, and possibly more healthy in the process, but they have no real desire to break world records, or be highly ranked among the triathlon set. And they don't want

**Table 1.1:** **Percentage of the population regarded as inactive or totally sedentary**

| | |
|---|---|
| Australia | 47%[4] |
| New Zealand | 49%[5] |
| United States | 66%[6] |
| United Kingdom | 48%[7] |

*Source:* Owen & Bauman (1992)[4]; Hillary Commission (1990)[5]; Public Health Service (1991)[6]; Allied Dunbar (1994)[7]

to miss out on too many of life's little luxuries to get rid of their excess body fat.

There's another reason why fitness and fatness are less correlated than thought in the past. Much of the traditional nutrition and exercise advice for increasing fitness is now no longer regarded as appropriate for fat loss. This knowledge has come about through research in the area of exercise physiology, down to the microcellular level, particularly since the early 1980s. The same has not yet happened in the body fat area and scientific knowledge on fat physiology is only just starting to accumulate.

## WHY FATNESS?

People working in the obesity area use the term *weight control*, and the measure of *weight* as their surrogate measurement of body fatness. Yet degree of fatness only partially contributes to body *weight*. Muscle tissue is almost two-and-a half times as dense as fat tissue and therefore a muscular person is likely to weigh more than a fat person of the same overall body size. Hence a fit, exercising person with a high muscle density is likely to weigh more, but have a much lower fat level than an unfit, fat person.

Weight is the combination of a range of things; bones, organs, muscle, even the length you grow your hair; whereas fat, if measured properly, is just fat. The difficulty, of course, is in accurate measurement. As you'll see in Chapter 6, there are no simple, accurate measurements for body fat. So far, there are only reasonable estimates. Still, these existing measurements are likely to give a better estimate of fatness level than the more general measure of body weight. A change in body weight, however, usually reflects changes in fat mass and lean mass (particularly in women), and hence the terms *weight* and *weight control*, while not technically correct, are still used as a form of convenience.

In this book, we have tried to use the terms *fat* and *overfatness* where this is a more accurate representation of the situation, except where referring to weight as such, or where this is used

5

to describe other work more specifically directed at weight. Despite their awkwardness, the terms *overfatness* and *fat control* are used where possible in an effort to get those working in this area to use the appropriate terminology. However, most studies, especially in larger populations, have to rely on some form of weight measurement as a surrogate for fatness.

## DEFINITIONS OF OVERWEIGHT AND OBESITY

The usual definition of *overfatness* or *overweight* is up to 20 per cent over a recognised ideal body weight[8], or a body mass index (BMI) (or height–weight measure see Chapter 3) of 25–29.9. BMI is a measure using weight divided by height squared $(kg/m^2)$; the normally recognised 'ideal' is a BMI of 20–25. *Obesity* is regarded here as a BMI of 30–39.9; and *morbid obesity* as BMI over 40. The levels used are shown in Table 1.2. While these categories do vary somewhat by different countries, the figures shown here are those used by the World Health Organisation (WHO).

## LEVELS OF FATNESS IN POPULATIONS

The prevalence of overfatness in the modern world is related to Westernisation. With industrialisation comes ease of accessibility to foods, especially processed and fatty foods. Some industrialised countries have a higher level of overall fatness than others, with Eastern Europeans currently topping the charts. The United States is at the top of the fatness tree amongst Western nations, but Australia, New Zealand and the United Kingdom are not far behind (see Table 1.3).

Fatness is even more prevalent in certain ethnic groups such as Australian Aborigines, Pacific Islanders and American Indians. It has been suggested that these people may have a genetic makeup ('thrifty genotype') which enables them to store more fat

**Table 1.2: WHO definitions of overweight and obesity**

| Category | Popular description | BMI |
|---|---|---|
| Underweight | Thin | <20.0 |
| Normal | Healthy weight | 20.0–24.9 |
| Grade I—Overweight | Moderate overweight | 25.0–29.9 |
| Grade II—Overweight | Obesity | 30.0–39.9 |
| Grade III—Overweight | Morbid obesity | >40.0 |

Source: WHO (1995)[9]

**Table 1.3: Overweight and obesity (as measured by BMI) in various countries***

| | Overweight | | Obese | |
|---|---|---|---|---|
| | Males (BMI >25–30) | Females (BMI >25–30) | Males (BMI >30) | Females (BMI >30) |
| Australia (1994) | 40% | 22% | 9% | 10% |
| Canada (1993) | 40% | 28% | 9% | 12% |
| New Zealand (1994) | 42% | 27% | 10% | 13% |
| UK (1994) | 42% | 25% | 12% | 15% |
| USA (1993) | 44% | 28% | 12% | 12% |

Note:* Figures estimated from a range of published sources

during times of 'feast' and/or use less energy during times of 'famine'. It is proposed that the harsh conditions and inconsistent food supply would have preferentially selected those people with the 'thrifty genotype' by giving them a survival advantage. To date, no genes have been found which endower a major propensity for fat storage and it seems unlikely that the genetic predisposition to obesity will be pinpointed to one or a few genes. Nor have any genetic markers for obesity been found in ethnic groups with high rates of obesity.

What is well known is that ethnic groups like the Aboriginal people suffer from a high rate of obesity-related diseases such as adult onset diabetes. In Nauru, for example, where super phosphate has made the population rich and the island poor, Professor Paul Zimmett of the WHO has estimated that around 20–30 per cent of the adult population have diabetes.[10] The Pima Indians of Arizona, who have been acculturated to the modern American diet, have extreme levels of obesity and the highest rate of diabetes in the world at 50 per cent of the adult population (compared to around 3 per cent in the White community).

This picture of an obese Western world might suggest that people are indifferent to their growing corpulence. Yet the figures show otherwise. Surveys carried out in the US suggest that at least 25 per cent of men and 40 per cent of women are trying to lose weight at any one time. Over the course of a year, the number of people who attempt to lose weight at least once rises to around 40 per cent for men and 80 per cent for women. The average man wants to lose 22kg to weigh 80kg and the average woman 22.5kg to weigh 60kg. Only 27 per cent of those who see themselves as overweight admit to not currently trying to slim. Perhaps as expected, the majority are using diet as the main method—76 per cent of men and 85 per cent of women. Around 60 per cent of both men and women use increased physical activity as a means of reducing weight.[11,12]

## REASONS FOR POPULATION INCREASES IN OBESITY

Exact reasons for the increases in fatness in the community are not as clear as they might seem to the layperson. Research has failed to provide conclusive evidence on any single factor and the evidence on a range of different factors (see Table 1.4), is often equivocal. For example, there is little to suggest that total energy consumption is the main culprit. Although obese people generally do consume more calories than lean people, there is still a wide variation between people. Also, active people are known to be big eaters but aren't necessarily fat. Athletes are the extreme example of this, but of course they are also highly active. As far as we can tell, people in most industrialised countries now consume around the same or less total energy intake as their grandparents, yet their grandparents didn't seem to have the same battle with the bulge. While there are significant problems assessing total energy intake, all indications are that this has not increased sufficiently to account for the increases in obesity now being seen.

Change in the *type* of food that's being eaten would seem to be the next obvious factor—fatty foods and fast foods in particular. Indeed, a correlation between fat consumption and obesity in some countries, like France, where the records have been available for years, would tend to support this. Since the turn of the century the percentage of fat in the diet has undoubtedly increased, but most of the increase has been in the last few decades. In countries like Australia, the UK and the US, the overall consumption of fat may have stabilised or even decreased. Sugar consumption doesn't seem to be related, as countries with high sugar consumption (e.g. Cuba) have low average body fat levels. Those with a high sugar consumption within countries are also amongst the leanest in a community, possibly because sugar and fat are generally inversely correlated. Large increases in soft drink and fruit juice consumption

**Table 1.4: Suggested causes of increased fatness in the community**

| Suggested cause | Supporting evidence |
| --- | --- |
| • Increased total energy intake | • Evidence suggests a decrease in intake |
| • Increased fat intake | • Little change or decrease |
| • Increased sugar intake | • Little change |
| • Increased soft drink intake | • Increases over 10 per cent per year |
| • Increased alcohol intake | • Actual decrease in many countries |
| • Increased variety/palatability of food | • No firm evidence but appears to be true |
| • Decreased work time activity | • Decreasing but contribution uncertain |
| • Decreased leisure time activity | • Probably increasing in some groups |
| • Decreased 'incidental' activity | • No data, but seems to be decreasing |
| • Decreased smoking rates | • Weight increasing in all smoking categories |

have occurred in recent years, however the connection between this and the increase in obesity is speculative only. Increases in alcohol are a further possibility, but consumption of this has generally been going down in those countries where obesity is increasing and consumption levels in populations often correlates inversely with obesity levels. In fact there's now little evidence to support the notion that alcohol *per se* is fattening.

Smoking rates are declining in most advanced countries, and it is known that the average smoker gains around 3kg over a 12-month period after quitting. Might this be a reason for increases in fatness at a community level? Several studies have shown that it may be a small contributor, but the increases in weight have been amongst smokers, ex-smokers and non-smokers, suggesting that it's not just quitters who have been the gainers.[13]

A more obvious, but still not statistically supported, association is the decline in physical activity levels. Although many people *claim* (from self reports) to be more physically active, the considered World Health Organisation view is that they could well be less active because any increase in leisure time activity may have been more than countered by the decrease in demand for physical labour as well as the decrease in incidental physical activity (the energy used to carry out day-to-day activities). Just getting from A to B requires less energy as technology and facilities improve by the year. Machine-power is replacing man-power and push-button technology is invading every part of daily life. Statistics on physical activity in most countries have not been kept to verify this assumption, but this hypothesis appears feasible. One finding, comparing the rise in obesity in the UK to the much lower rise in the Netherlands, who have a similar dietary composition, claims that the fact that 27 per cent of the Dutch use bicycles as a means of transport compared to only 3 per cent of the English may provide some explanation.[14]

In the absence of evidence incriminating specific factors, it appears clear that increases in obesity are due to several changes in the recent human environment which allows the biological functions of fat to favour storage. Fatness obviously has an important survival function: it enables us to store energy to help get through the bad times. But like a lot of biological functions there is a range of healthy fat deposits, above and below which there is no longer any survival value, and illness occurs. It's really only in the last three decades or less that overfatness has become so commonplace.

In Australia, since regular records have been kept from 1981, there has been a steady growth of around 0.7 per cent per year in the percentage of the population regarded as overweight or obese using a measure of BMI. This is similar to the increase in the US measured by the National Health and Nutrition Examination Surveys (NHANES) carried out at regular intervals.[15] There appears also to be a faster rate of growth in the extreme categories of fatness and in lower socioeconomic (SE) groups. Obesity in Australia for example, has doubled in the last decade with around 10 per cent of Australians now regarded as obese. The majority of these are from lower SE groups. The Australian Institute of Health estimates that around 5 million Australians are now overfat (including the more severe category of obesity). In North America and Europe the estimate is 50 and 100 million respectively. This has led National Heart Foundations in the Western world to be concerned about reversals of gains made in heart disease prevention through increases in obesity.

## GENETIC VERSUS ENVIRONMENTAL EFFECTS

Clearly both the environment and genetics are responsible for obesity, but how do they inter-relate? There are large differences in the amount of obesity between populations. Some of this variation can be explained by differences in body frame which makes it difficult to compare, for example, Samoans with Cambodians. However, even within Caucasian populations there is a wide range in the percentage of people who are obese. In many Eastern European countries, about 30–45 per cent of females would be classified as obese compared with about 10–13 per cent in Australia and New Zealand. These differences in the prevalence of obesity are largely dependent on differences in the environment (fat

**Figure 1.1: Genetic influence on obesity in the Pima Indians of Arizona**

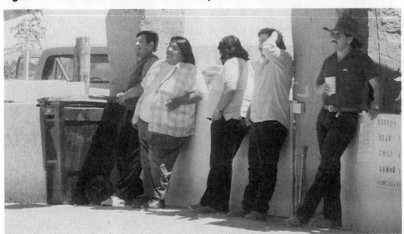

content of the typical diet, food variety and availability, and availability of labour-saving devices). This is also shown by the increases in obesity within a population over time and in ethnic groups who migrate from 'low obesity' to 'high obesity' countries.

Within any particular environment, however, the response of individuals to that environment will vary. Some may respond to a high fat diet with only a small gain in weight, whereas others will gain a lot. How much an individual responds to the environment is largely dependent on his or her genetic makeup. The most convincing evidence for this has come from a series of studies performed by Dr Claude Bouchard and others from Laval University in Quebec, on identical twins. They increased the calorie intake of twins by 1000kcal/day for 3 months under strictly controlled conditions. Naturally, everyone gained weight, but some gained much more than others. If one twin only gained a few kilograms, the other twin tended to have a small weight gain as well. If one twin gained a lot of weight, so did the other twin. In other words, under identical environmental conditions, people gain weight at different rates and the amount they gain seems to be genetically determined[16] (see Figure 1.2).

This can be viewed in another way using the population distribution of body size (Figure 1.3). Consider a population that lives in an environment which does not promote obesity—such as a remote Pacific island with little contact with the outside world, where the food has to be gathered, and where deep-fried chicken is still unknown (environment A). There will be a variety of body sizes, but very few will be classified as obese. Then an airport is

**Figure 1.2:   Weight gain in identical twins after 3 months overfeeding**

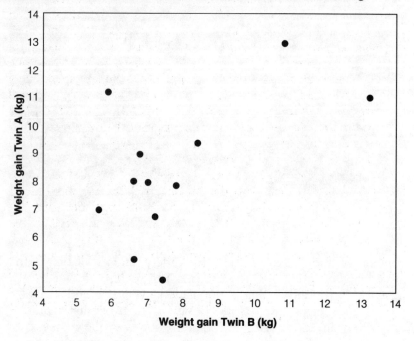

**Figure 1.3:   Distribution of body fatness in the community**

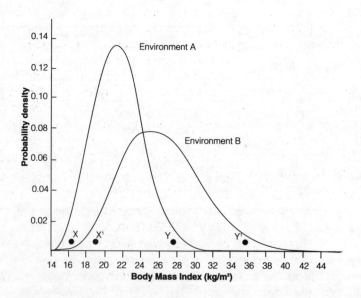

built, the tourists arrive, motorised transport takes over from legs and paddles and the fried chicken takeaways set up business. Ten years later, the population distribution of body size has shifted to the right and more people are now classified as obese (environment B). However, the distribution is skewed, so not everyone gained weight at the same rate. A person X who is 'genetically lean' and is at the left hand side of the curve gained only a small amount of weight as the environment changed from A to B. Person Y happens to be genetically more predisposed to weight gain and is on the right hand side of the curve. He or she gained considerable weight and in environment B is now obese (Y¹).

This shift in population levels of obesity also provides evidence for approaches to deal with the problem. Individual, one-on-one approaches (the 'high risk' approach) are obviously necessary. But these do little to affect the total population. A small shift in the total curve shown in Figure 1.3 to the left on the other hand, will have a major effect on public health. In other words, small fat losses in a large number of people will have a greater impact on the health of the population as a whole than larger losses in a small number. This is the public health approach to obesity considered more in Chapter 7.

## CHANGES IN THINKING ABOUT OBESITY AND OVERFATNESS

While fatness has never been highly regarded in modern societies, and while there has been a weight control industry around for some time to cater for people with cosmetic concerns, the real interest in fatness—as a health issue—is relatively new. It began in the 1950s with the discovery that a high body weight and abdominal fat were related to a number of diseases. Our understanding of these factors has increased in recent years with a growing awareness of the extent of the problem. Table 1.5 shows some of the changes in thinking that have occurred in that time.

The most significant changes have occurred in our understanding of measures of body fatness, what causes fatness and appropriate treatment and prevention strategies.

### MYTH-INFORMATION
*'Passive' exercise devices, by definition, can have no effect on fat loss. A basic principle is '. . . if you don't work, neither does the machine'.*

**Table 1.5:   Changes in thinking about overfatness and obesity**

|  | 1980s | 1990s |
|---|---|---|
| Measures | • Weight, BMI, Skinfolds | • Machine measures<br>• Fat distribution |
| Causes | • Excess total calories<br>• Lack of exercise | • Fat calories<br>• Physical inactivity<br>• Genetic influences<br>• Environment |
| Other | • Limited health risk<br>• Small sex differences | • Major health risk<br>• Big sex differences |
| Treatment | • Dieting<br>• Vigorous exercise | • Lifestyle change<br>• Moderate physical activity |

Ideas about measuring fat have shifted with changes in technology, and we have a better understanding of the types and distribution of fat related to disease. In general there has been a shift away from a single fat measure towards a combination, including body mass index, sagittal diameter and waist circumference, that can be used in a practical situation. Technological advances have meant that new, portable machines, such as Bio-impedance Analysis (BIA) and Near Infrared Analysis (NIR) have become accessible and of some value to the non-expert user. At the 'high tech' end, expensive devices such as Dual Energy X-Ray Absorptiometry (DEXA), Magnetic Resonance Imaging (MRI), Computerised Tomography (CT) and Ultrasound have now all but taken over from the 'gold standard' of underwater weighing to image fat mass proportions. All of these measures are discussed in detail in Chapter 6.

The main changes in thinking about the causes of overfatness centre around the type, rather than quantity of food eaten (e.g. the influence of energy from fat on total energy), and the impact of individual factors (particularly genetics) in influencing body fatness. There are, for example, big genetic differences in fat gain and in the extent of fat loss in response to a particular exercise or diet stimulus, and these have not been sufficiently recognised in the past. The interaction of biology with the environment and behaviour also needs to be considered. Understanding the causes of fatness is, of course, vital to the development of correct techniques of coping with it. The implications of all these changes for those interested in fat loss or maintenance of body fat are quite new. They are discussed in some length throughout the rest of this book.

Other changes in orientation have included a re-analysis of

the role of fatness in ill-health. Epidemiological studies carried out in the 1960s and 1970s found little correlation between weight and major diseases like heart disease, because the measure of fatness used was generally a measure of body mass (i.e. weight or body mass index (BMI)), which discriminates against healthy, lean, muscular individuals. Epidemiological studies also looked for independent effects of obesity, whereas its effects are largely mediated via other risk factors such as high blood pressure. A re-analysis of these data has now shown that fat distribution is a key factor in ill-health and this explains much of the earlier epidemiological evidence (Chapter 2). It's not only *if* someone is fat that is important in health terms, but also *where* they are fat.

There has also been an increasing emphasis on gender, race and age and other individual factors on fat gain and loss, to the extent that it's becoming apparent that any program must be individualised, as stressed throughout this book. However, recognition of the importance of the environment also makes a public health approach imperative.

There has also been a change away from the concentration on 'diet' as a form of treatment towards a change in lifestyle which, unlike short term diets, can be maintained over a lifetime. This includes a move away from exercise designed for cardiovascular fitness, towards an increase in the level of total activity—both planned and 'incidental'—that is carried out within our changing, modern technological lifestyles. To this extent, professionals who deal only in prescribing diets or exercise are unlikely to maintain a primary role in fat loss through lifestyle management in the future. These issues are covered in detail in the sections on exercise in Chapters 12 and 13.

Finally, a major shift in direction, begun in the 1990s, has been a change in thinking about the psychological aspects of obesity and body fat maintenance. In the 1970s, the use of behaviour modification techniques in weight control began and this has now become standard in most modern programs. More recently it's been recognised that much more complex, emotional and cognitive (thinking) functions are involved in obesity. This is particularly so in the case of many women, who have suffered much more social and psychological pressure than men to attain an unrealistic body shape, and as a result have often developed counter-productive cognitive cycles of guilt, depression and anger associated with food and food restriction. Modern approaches need to pay more attention to dealing with these issues. Counselling also needs to become more reflective and less directive to empower people to resolve these issues themselves rather than simply replace one dependency (food) with another (a counsellor).

## A NEW PARADIGM FOR WEIGHT CONTROL

All this suggests that the area of weight control is going through a major paradigm shift. The older, simplistic notions of 'change in weight = energy in (food) – energy out (exercise)', are no longer applicable. On the food side of the equation, there has been a shift away from total energy, or total calories, as being solely important, to a greater emphasis on the importance of dietary fat. Energy balance has thus become 'fat balance' and 'dieting' has given way to food planning and lifestyle eating patterns. Similarly, the role of vigorous, organised exercise has given way to a greater emphasis on fat use through longer duration, lower intensity activity, along with an increase in the type of 'incidental movement' that can be added to daily life.

The environment, biology and behaviour are also vital in any assessment of causes, and whilst these are mediated through the energy balance equation, no detailed discussion of fat loss man-agement can be considered without them. Finally, more account needs to be taken of the body's physiological adjustment mecha-nisms. Static equations relating to energy intake and energy expenditure which do not consider the dynamic adjustment of the body to changes in body composition and energy balance are no longer realistic. A more appropriate paradigm would attempt to take account of these adjustments. Hence, the old 'physics' style weight control paradigm is slowly giving way to a new, more personalised 'ecological' approach. In Chapter 7, after examining the health and physiological effects of fat and how it is measured, we spell out such a paradigm for use in the practical situation. The remainder of the book is then centred around explaining the components of this paradigm and their implications for dealing with overfatness and obesity.

## IMPLICATIONS

1. Whatever is being done to reduce obesity is not working and the developed world will be facing an explosion of diabetes and other diseases if obesity continues to increase.
2. Programs to decrease fatness should be markedly different to programs to increase fitness.

3. Body weight is only a surrogate measure of fatness and the term 'overfatness' should be used where possible.
4. The aetiology of obesity is complex and it is particularly important to work closely with specialists when dealing with the severely obese.
5. Obesity and overfatness have complex, multi-factorial causes with biological, environmental and behavioural determinants suggesting that any notion of these being due to sloth or gluttony alone are now outdated.
6. Obese individuals need to understand that their degree of overfatness is genetically determined to a significant degree and that achieving a slim body requires a lifelong swim against the twin adverse tides of genes and environment. Realistic fat loss goals need to be set.
7. A population needs to change its environment to reduce the prevalence of obesity. Even small changes spread across the whole population have major influences.
8. There is a need to re-orient thinking about weight control from a simplistic, energy balance approach to a more complex, multi-dimensional, holistic approach involving long term life-style modification.

# 2
# Fat in health and disease

## SUMMARY OF MAIN POINTS

- Fat has a variety of functions, but the most important is as an energy reserve. A minimum level of body fat is essential for this purpose.
- Excessive body fat can have disease implications.
- The health implications of obesity are determined by total fat and fat distribution.
- Visceral fat, or fat stored around the organs of the trunk, is the most dangerous to health.
- Abdominal fat, or a 'pot belly', is the most visible indication of visceral fat.
- Diabetes, heart disease, gallstones and some cancers are the main diseases associated with excessive abdominal fatness.

## WHAT IS FAT?

Fat is a highly valuable substance which exists in some form in many plants, seeds and animals. In plants and seeds, it is mainly stored in the form of oils. In humans and animals it's stored in body tissue known as *adipose tissue*, which is made up of many fat cells or *adipocytes*. The main types of fats in plants and animals are called *triglycerides*. The main function of the fat cell is as a storage reserve of these triglycerides for energy, but it also has secondary functions of providing a 'cushion' or protection for the organs of the body and insulating against heat loss. Before it gets into the fat cell, fat in the bloodstream also acts as a transport medium for fat-soluble vitamins such as vitamins A, D, E and K.

While triglycerides are the main type of fat used by the body, two other fats, cholesterol and phospholipids, also have important functions. Cholesterol is a waxy fat-like substance which is used for the production of certain substances such as sex hormones, and in the structure of cell membranes (cell lining). The phospholipids make up part of the structure of every cell, particularly the cell membrane. In our diet, almost all of the fat is in the form of triglycerides with only a small amount of cholesterol and phospholipids.

---

**Functions of fat in the body**

- Energy reserve (i.e. 1g of fat = 9kcal of energy).
- Protection of the vital organs (e.g. stomach, kidneys, liver etc).
- Heat insulation.
- Transport medium for fat-soluble vitamins and minerals (e.g. vitamins D, E and K).
- Formation of hormones (e.g. cholesterol).
- Structure of cell membranes (cholesterol and phospholipids).

---

## THE SURVIVAL VALUE OF FAT

Because of its efficiency as an energy store, fat has traditionally had great survival value in humans. This has been shown many times in survival situations such as shipwrecks or plane crashes. The person with the higher percentage of body fat is more likely to survive under conditions of food deprivation.

The higher percentage of body fat in (pre-menopausal) females serves the biological function of helping to preserve the species in situations of famine. If women lose too much fat they become amenorrhoeic (don't ovulate and therefore do not have periods) and thus are not able to conceive.

Fat is the highest source of food energy that can be obtained (9kcal/g compared with 4.5kcal/g for carbohydrate or protein), so fatty foods would have had survival value in a hunter-gatherer environment. According to Professor Kerin O'Dea from Deakin University[1] this may explain our taste for fatty foods which still persists today. Unfortunately (or fortunately, depending on your point of view), there is now no shortage of available fat, particularly from processed foods. There is also no need to expend so much energy (and therefore 'burn off' fat) by having to chase our food. So, for the first time in human history, people can over-indulge their biological liking for fat, under-indulge their physical activity requirements—and get fat in the process.

## Total body mass and health

Overfatness has typically been inferred from measures of body mass, such as weight or body mass index (see Chapter 3). Mass is not always a good measure of fatness, because of the influence of muscle and other lean body tissue. However, measures of body mass index (BMI) still show a correlation with disease risk, and particularly mortality levels, or the risks of premature death. Mortality levels have a 'tick-shaped' association with BMI (Figure 2.1) with the highest risks of mortality at increasing levels of obesity over a BMI of 25. There is also a slightly increased risk of mortality at BMI levels below 20, which is largely explained by the presence of existing disease and smoking, both of which are causes of lower weight and higher mortality.

The relative risk of various diseases with increased obesity levels (as measured by BMI) are shown in Table 2.1. Relative risk (RR) is an indication of the proportional increase in risk of disease from a standard measure of 1.0. Hence, a RR of 2.0 means the risk of contracting that disease is twice that of someone with a normal BMI.

### FAT AS A PRIMARY HEALTH RISK

Fat, as we've seen, is vital for existence. However, as is often the case, too much of a good thing can be dangerous. Health experts have long known the problems of overfatness, but it has often been under-rated as a *primary* health risk, partly because BMI is only a blunt measure of fatness. Fat distribution as well as total fatness is of critical importance. European researchers have known this for some time since the famous French endocrinologist Jean Vague published it in 1956.[3] More recently, North American and European researchers have gone back and re-examined the epidemiological data using measures of fat distribution such as

**Figure 2.1: Mortality risk by extent of obesity (as measured by BMI)**

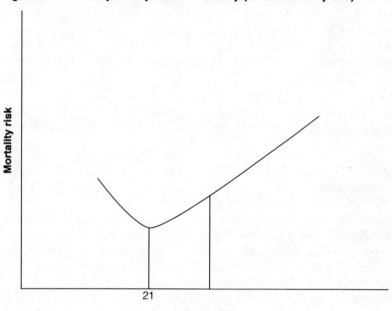

**Body Mass Index**

**Table 2.1: Relative risk of selected conditions for obese people**

|                              | Relative risk (RR) |
| ---------------------------- | ------------------ |
| Diabetes (NIDDM)[a]          | 16.7               |
| Gallstones                   | 10.0               |
| Coronary heart disease       | 3.3                |
| Hypertension                 | 4.3                |
| Breast cancer[b]             | 1.3                |
| Colon cancer                 | 1.3                |

*Note:* [a] Non insulin dependent diabetes mellitus
      [b] Post-menopausal women only
*Source:* Colditz (1992)[2]

waist-to-hip ratio (WHR) instead of weight, and found that *abdominal* fatness (i.e. a 'pot belly') is just as powerful and important a primary risk factor in determining ill-health as other risk factors such as high cholesterol, high blood pressure and smoking in causing problems such as heart disease, late onset or non insulin dependent diabetes mellitus (NIDDM) and some forms of cancer.[4]

## BODY FAT DISTRIBUTION

The location of fat on an individual's body is partly due to genetic

**Figure 2.2:    The three main fat shapes**

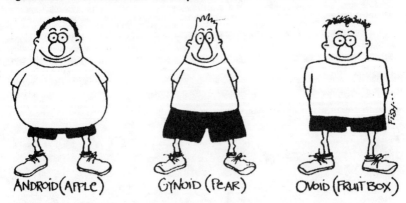

ANDROID (APPLE)          GYNOID (PEAR)          OVOID (FRUIT BOX)

influences, but is also idiosyncratic. Some people store fat on the upper body, some on the lower body; some get fat around the neck first, some around the arms and chest. In general, men store fat around the waist or abdomen, and pre-menopausal women store fat around the hips and buttocks.[5] These are the typical *android* (apple) and *gynoid* (pear) shapes that distinguish men and women. A third, generally 'big all over' shape, is the *ovoid* (fruit box) form of overfatness. This is often more characteristic of those with a genetic predisposition to obesity. The three classical types of fat shapes are shown in Figure 2.2.

An analysis of national figures in the United Kingdom shows that while the 'apple' and 'pear' are the majority shapes of males and females respectively, around 14 per cent of men may be fat and pear-shaped and 27 per cent of women fat and apple-shaped.[6] This is perhaps not unexpected with women because at menopause they lose the benefits of the female hormones, particularly oestrogen, which maintain female fat in the lower body (hips, thighs and buttocks) for reproductive purposes, and they begin to store more fat on the upper body, like men. Increases in abdominal fat in men and women differ with age, as can be seen in Figure 2.3. Women, in general, tend to store more fat around the lower regions until they reach menopause. Then they put it on like men. Men, on the other hand, generally increase their abdominal stores linearly with age from around 25 years on.

FAT DISTRIBUTION AND HEALTH

The apple shape has been found to be much more potentially dangerous with respect to health than the pear shape, because

**Figure 2.3: Abdominal fat by age and sex**

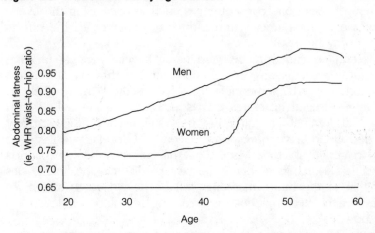

the fat cells around the abdomen release their fat into the bloodstream more readily than other fat cells. A 'pot belly' therefore—irrespective of total body mass—is likely to be more *atherogenic* (i.e. cause narrowing of the arteries), *diabetogenic* (i.e. cause diabetes) and possibly *carcinogenic* (i.e. cause cancer). In contrast, pear-shaped women have been found to have little increased illness risk (with the possible exception of a slight increase in the risk of varicose veins and arthritis). In health terms therefore, it's not *if* someone is fat, but *where* they are fat that is important—filling up of the fat cells around the waist (as is characteristic of men) is much more dangerous than filling up of fat cells on the lower body (as is more characteristic of women).[7]

There is another important form of fat storage not shown in Figure 2.2 which is now thought to be most important as a predictor of ill-health. *Visceral fat* (sometimes called 'intra-abdominal fat'), surrounds the organs or 'viscera' of the body, such as the stomach, liver and kidneys etc. Visceral fat is thought to be dangerous because it 'gives up' its fat into the *portal circulation*

---

MYTH-INFORMATION

*Although there are identified body fat shapes with varying health risks, there is no evidence that specific diets have special effects for any one particular body shape, hence there is no support for a 'body shape' diet.*

---

in the bloodstream, which passes through the liver first. This has a variety of metabolic consequences such as increasing the liver's production of fat particles and inducing resistance to the effects of the hormone insulin.[8]

Visceral fat can only be seen using special medical imaging techniques but it is also highly correlated with total abdominal fat. In other words, someone with a 'pot belly' is more likely to have large visceral fat stores than someone who has a low level of total abdominal fat—although it is still possible for relatively lean people to have quite high visceral fat levels, possibly due again to genetic factors. Visceral fat has recently been explained by health researchers as being the best predictor of health risk. It's likely that in the future measures will be developed to screen for this in health check-ups, just as screening for blood cholesterol is done now.

Table 2.2 summarises the fat storage types and their associated health risks.

The health risks of fat shapes is illustrated in Figure 2.4 which combines both BMI (body mass index) and WHR (waist-to-hip ratio) measures. As can be seen, it's not just the big person who is at risk. A small person with large abdominal fat stores (i.e. a 'pot belly' is also at risk).

**Table 2.2: Health risks and characteristics of fat shapes**

| Fat type | Identifying shape | Most common in | CVD[1] | NIDDM[2] | Cancers | Arthritis | Varicose veins |
|---|---|---|---|---|---|---|---|
| Visceral fat | Mainly android but could be any of the below | Android shaped males | +++ | +++ | + | ? | – |
| Android | 'Apple' shaped | Men and post-menopausal women | + | + | + | ? | – |
| Gynoid | 'Pear' shaped | Pre-menopausal women | – | – | – | ? | ? |
| Ovoid | 'Fruit box' shaped | Men and women but more genetic and of longer origin | + | + | ? | + | + |

*Notes:* 1 Cardiovascular disease
2 Non insulin dependent diabetes mellitus
+++ = Very high risk   ++ = High risk   + = Some risk
? = Risk not known but suspected

**Figure 2.4: Fat shapes and health risks**

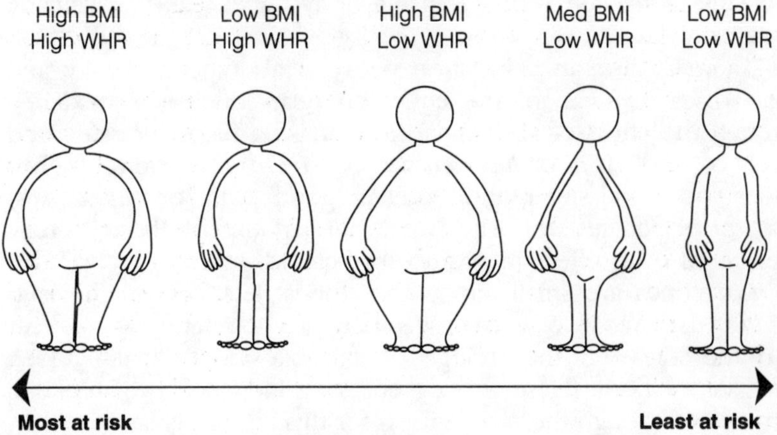

| High BMI<br>High WHR | Low BMI<br>High WHR | High BMI<br>Low WHR | Med BMI<br>Low WHR | Low BMI<br>Low WHR |
|---|---|---|---|---|

**◄ Most at risk**      **Least at risk ►**

**Figure 2.5: Health problems associated with overfatness**

| Disease | Risk Factors | Less Obvious |
|---|---|---|
| Diabetes | Blood pressure | Back problems |
| Gallstones | Cholesterol | Snoring/OSA |
| Bowel cancer | Blood sugars | EDS |
| Heart disease | | Knee problems |
| Post-menopausal | | Skin problems |
| breast cancer | | Sex problems |
| | Sydnrome X | Psycho-social problems |

Note: OSA Obstructive sleep apnoea
    EDS Excessive daytime sleepiness

## DISEASE ASSOCIATIONS

As well as diseases, there are a number of other health problems associated with obesity, particularly abdominal obesity. These are listed in Figure 2.5.

The association of abdominal obesity with adult diabetes is an important one as the incidence is rising in the population in proportion to the rise in obesity levels. In the early 1970s, around 1 per cent of the population in Australia suffered from diabetes. By the mid 1990s that had risen to 3 per cent and is predicted to be closer to 5 per cent by the turn of the century, giving medical authorities concern about diabetes as a major epidemic of the future. It is estimated that around 80–90 per cent of all adult onset diabetes (in contrast to childhood onset, or insulin dependent diabetes) is associated with obesity, particularly abdominal obesity. The exact cause is not clear, but the progression from insulin resistance to *hyperinsulinaemia* (high blood insulin) to *hyperglycaemia* (high blood sugar) and then full blown diabetes, is clearly associated with increasing body fatness, and particularly abdominal fatness.

There is also an association between abdominal obesity and heart disease. Some of the effect on heart disease is mediated through the effect of abdominal fat in raising blood pressure and levels of 'bad' (LDL or *low density lipoprotein*) cholesterol, triglycerides and blood sugar, and reducing 'good' (HDL or *high density lipoprotein*) cholesterol. However, independent of these factors, there is also an effect in promoting heart disease.

Gallstones are small, crystalline stones that form in the gallbladder as a result of excess secretion of cholesterol by the liver into the bile and the storage of the bile in the gall-bladder. Excesses of body fat seem to predispose individuals to gallstone formation although the mechanisms for this are not clear. Similarly, there is an association between obesity and bowel cancer and post-menopausal breast cancer, although again the mechanisms are presently not well understood.

As well as these diseases, abdominal fat has been associated with an increase in disease risk factors such as high blood pressure, high blood sugar and an abnormal pattern of blood fats (low HDL cholesterol and high triglycerides). Together with these three indicators, abdominal fatness combines to form a condition now known as 'syndrome X', the 'metabolic syndrome', or 'the deadly quartet', which is known to be highly predictive of a range of diseases including heart disease and diabetes.[9] It has been proposed that abdominal fatness is actually the cause of 'syndrome X'—abdominal fat leads to increased fatty acids in the blood and insulin resistance, which then leads to the other three in the quartet—high blood sugars, high blood fats and high blood pressure.[10]

OTHER HEALTH PROBLEMS ASSOCIATED WITH OVERFATNESS

There is also a range of other less obvious problems associated with obesity, and particularly abdominal obesity. One of these is obstructive sleep apnoea (OSA).[11] OSA is an interruption to sleep caused by blockages to the windpipe producing breathing disruption. The problem is often characterised by heavy snoring. Typically, there is a period of snoring followed by a short period of silence when the breathing ceases and then it starts again with a stutter. The apnoea (lack of breathing) occurs when the person enters the deepest stage of sleep and the tongue relaxes, obstructing the airway.

**Figure 2.6: The sleep apnoea/abdominal fatness cycle**

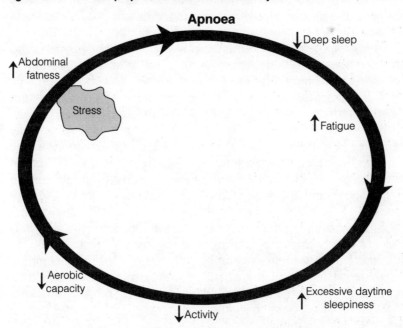

Apnoea

↓ Deep sleep

↑ Abdominal fatness

Stress

↑ Fatigue

↓ Aerobic capacity

↓ Activity

↑ Excessive daytime sleepiness

Obesity is often associated with increased fat deposition in the tongue and throat structures and this can cause the airway obstruction in many sleep apnoea sufferers. Reducing body fat— even by as little as 10 per cent in some people—can reduce the problems of OSA. OSA is most common in men and has a direct role in injury, particularly in the workplace. Disruption of the deepest stage of sleep at night can lead to excessive daytime sleepiness (EDS), which results in a vicious cycle of reduced exercise capacity, stress, over-eating and hence an even greater level of obesity (Figure 2.6). Daytime tiredness is now known to increase the risk of injury; truck drivers with OSA are now banned from driving in some countries.

In many instances of OSA it may be necessary to improve sleep patterns before the patient has sufficient daytime energy to break the cycle and carry out physical activity which can lead to fat loss. Devices such as a constant peak airways pressure (CPAP) machine, which keeps the breathing passage open by maintaining a positive pressure in the airways, can be valuable. Although dealing only with symptoms, this allows a patient to feel rested and suffer less excessive daytime sleepiness and thus perhaps to be more active during the day, potentially decreasing the overfatness which caused the problem.

Joint problems, such as knee pain, are also common in very big people. This is because of the extra pressure put on the joints by carrying excessive weight. Often this can be a limiting factor in getting big people to exercise. However, it's not uncommon to find that these problems improve on a fat reduction program as the individual begins to lose fat, and hence some body weight.

Skin infections can be a further problem. A fungal infection called *intertrigo* which causes itchiness and a rash, can flourish in the hot, damp environment under the 'apron', or fold of belly fat in very big people. Fungal infections are also common on the insteps of the feet, which often never see the light of day, because of the extra weight forcing them into and against the inner surface of the shoes and the heat created by synthetic socks and leather shoes. This is one reason why big men often insist on wearing 'thongs' or sandals which air the feet, without knowing that it is their obesity which is causing the problem. *Tinea pedis*, an infection between the toes or under the feet, is also more common in fat men because of the hot and sweaty micro-environment of the feet. *Pitted keralysis* is a bubbling form of rash under the soles of the feet, also common in the obese, which causes the feet to smell. Regular washing only aggravates the problem as this reduces the skin's natural oiliness and dries it out even more. Regular airing by wearing open shoes or punching holes in the insteps of shoes with a nail punch can help overcome the problem. *Acanthosis nigrocans* is another skin problem, characterised by velvety, pigmented patches around the underarms, sides of the trunk, knuckles and groin. Acanthosis is occasionally a sign of severe insulin resistance.

Finally, sexual difficulties and psycho-social problems can also result from excessive body fatness. In relation to sexual difficulties, poor self-esteem, lack of fitness and lack of flexibility all combine to make this a significant psychological problem. Recent research has also shown that abdominal fatness in men is associated with a decrease in testosterone levels. This is quite contrary to the notion of a 'pot belly' being a proxy indication of manhood. Other psycho-social problems come from the widespread prejudice against fatness. Obese people are often judged to be lacking willpower and to be lazy, over-indulgent and stupid; fatness is strongly associated with ugliness.

All in all, there are few advantages in carrying excessive body fat in this modern day. Of course, the natural evolutionary advantage is the survival value that fat has in circumstances of reduced energy availability. In women, carrying around extra fat is associated with one health advantage, which is a reduction in the long term risk of osteoporosis. Bone appears to respond to the load it has to carry by becoming stronger. Beyond this, there is little real advantage in carrying body fat beyond the 25 and 30 per cent of total body mass recommended as the upper limits for males and females respectively.

---

### MYTH-INFORMATION

*'Negative calories' is a term used in some diets to suggest fat burning properties of food. There are no such things as negative calories and no 'fat burning' foods.*

---

## HEALTH EFFECTS OF WEIGHT CYCLING

Although there are major health consequences of overfatness and obesity, most people who lose body fat through organised diet and exercise plans often regain most of this within a few years; this pattern of weight cycling may continue throughout life. Weight cycling has received much attention in recent times because of reports that it may increase the risks of coronary heart disease.[12] These reports suggest that it may be more dangerous to lose and regain fat in a period of cycles than it is to be permanently fat.

However, evidence for the dangerous effects of weight cycling may have been exaggerated. Reviews of all the research in the area have led Professor Claude Bouchard and Professor Robert Jeffries, both experts in the area of obesity, to conclude that there is no real evidence that weight cycling is more dangerous to health than not reducing body fat. The severity and frequency of cycling may be the important issue to consider here.[13]

## IMPLICATIONS

1. People at risk for obesity-related health problems, especially adult onset diabetes, need to be particularly careful about gaining abdominal fat.
2. When assessing the health importance of obesity for an individual, total fat, fat distribution and risk of disease all need to be considered.
3. It is more crucial for abdominally obese people to reduce fat for health reasons than for people with a more gynoid pattern.

4. The primary location of fat storage in an individual (i.e. upper or lower body) influences not only the health risk but also the degree to which changes can be made in body fat content. Abdominal body fat stores tend to be more mobile than those in the lower body.
5. For this reason, body fat in android-shaped males is likely to be more easily mobilised than in most gynoid-shaped females.
6. Because of possible significant genetic, psychological and metabolic differences, long term cases of severe and morbid obesity should be regarded differently to short term cases of overfatness.
7. Because of hormonal changes, the fat loss response of post-menopausal women may be different to that of younger women and hence fat loss treatments may need to be different.
8. The genetic contribution to overfatness needs to be assessed to help determine the difficulty of the potential fat loss response.
9. Look for and consider less obvious health problems that may be related to excessive overfatness, e.g. bad back, bad knees, poor sleep, all of which may affect the fat loss response.
10. Be sensitive to psycho-social problems and sexual disorders in people who are excessively fat.
11. Accept that there are many factors influencing body fat and body shape that cannot be significantly modified, i.e. genetics, gender, age.

# II
# PHYSIOLOGY

# 3
# Fat physiology

SUMMARY OF MAIN POINTS

- Fat cells are similar to other cells, but contain a lipid or fat pool for storage of fats to be used as energy.
- The average human body has 30–50 billion fat cells, and obese people have up to 100 billion.
- Most increases in fat mass are associated with increases in fat cell size.
- *Lipogenesis* refers to the storage of fat in fat cells; *lipolysis* the breakdown of fat.
- Lipogenesis and lipolysis are controlled by a number of enzymes and hormones.
- There is a constant cycle of fat storage and breakdown at the fat cell level, but increases in lipolysis do not translate into increases in fat burning.
- The state of energy balance is the major influence in the lipogenesis/lipolysis cycle.

## THE FAT CELL

A fat cell (*adipocyte*) is similar in form to many other types of body cells with the exception of its storage 'depot'—a *lipid* (fat) pool, which can make up to 90 per cent of the cell (see Figure 3.1). Otherwise, the adipocyte has a cell nucleus, with all the

**Figure 3.1:   The human fat cell**

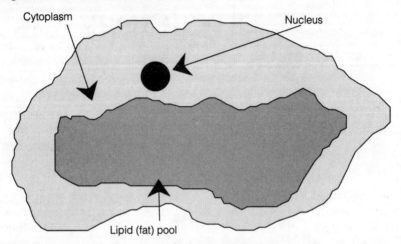

Cytoplasm

Nucleus

Lipid (fat) pool

'head office' functions and genetic materials of other cells, and the *cytoplasm* (the 'jelly') and *mitochondria* (the 'powerhouse') characteristic of skin, bone and other organ cells.

The average fat cell stores around 0.5 micrograms of fat in its lipid pool (a microgram is a millionth of a gram) and the average, non obese individual has between 30–50 billion of these fat cells throughout his/her body (in fact more on her than him, as you'll see below). Doing the sums on this, you can see that the average person will be carrying around 15kg of fat as his/her 'spare tank', or energy reserve.[1]

## FAT GAINS AND LOSSES

Fat is either gained or lost by increases or decreases in the size of the lipid pool in large numbers of fat cells. These 'fill up' in good times, like a water tank after heavy rain, and 'empty out' in bad times, like in a drought.

Which cells fill up or empty out most, and in what order, is a function of a range of factors including genetics, gender, age, race and the number of existing fat cells. One thing is clear though: the last cells to fill up are likely to be the first to empty out. If someone gains extra fat around the waist for example, this will usually be the first place it goes from when the energy balance becomes negative.

Fat cell enlargement through expansion of existing cells is called *hypertrophy*. A less common way of increasing fat is through an expansion of fat cell numbers or *hyperplasia*. Hyperplasia is thought to occur only at certain periods in life, in particular during growth spurts when all body cells are rapidly increasing in number, such as early infancy (1–2 years) and early adolescence (12–14 years). Inappropriate lifestyles at these times may lead to a greater increase in fat cell numbers than might otherwise occur. A third stimulus to hyperplasia which is now well recognised is a large increase in body fat. As existing fat cells 'fill up', new cells come into existence and form a bigger 'maximum capacity' which is then capable of storing a total greater volume of fat. In contrast to the 30–50 billion fat cells of the average person, an obese person may have 70–80 or even up to 100 billion adipocytes.

The basis for hyperplasia of fat cells consists of 'baby' fat cells, known as *adipocyte precursors*, which exist amongst other fat cells, as if waiting for the opportunity to spring into action and fill up with fat like their parent cells (see Figure 3.2).[2]

Not a lot is known about these precursors; whether they are actually small fat cells in waiting, or whether they are just other (*'stem'*) cells that can be called on to make any other form of cell if needed. Some research suggests that they spring into action during the growth spurts mentioned above if conditions are right, or when increases in body weight exceed around 170 per cent of ideal or average weight. Once they mature however, they are there for life. Animal research has shown that with severe dietary restriction, fat cells can shrink to the point where they are virtually unrecognisable as adipocytes, but when overfeeding begins again, the shrunken cells rapidly fill up with fat.

With the expansion of fat cells in the waist region, some men, in particular, develop a 'hard' fat belly and some a 'soft' or 'wobbly' fat one. The reasons for this are not quite clear but it's possible that the big, hard abdomen represents a larger degree of visceral fat within the abdomen, which then pushes out more on the inner

MYTH-INFORMATION

*Creams, rubs and lotions designed to get rid of cellulite do not work. Cellulite, which is a concocted name for groups of fat cells with less efficient connective tissue, responds like other fat cells. However, there is a genetic component which makes cellulite more common in some people (mainly women).*

**Figure 3.2: Fat cells and precursors**

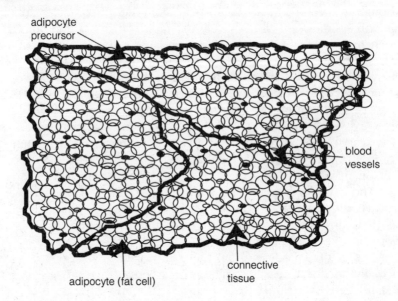

surface of the abdomen. Fat which is more 'wobbly' may represent more subcutaneous fat, although the evidence for this is not currently clear.

Irrespective of the type of fat stored, it's clear that it is easier to prevent obesity and overfatness beyond a certain level than to cure it. Obviously, the function of fat as an energy store means that the human body has a certain capacity for increases and decreases in fat stores without permanent change. In the long term and for the very obese, however, there may be more permanent changes in fat cell numbers, metabolism and other fat maintaining factors, which make it more difficult to reduce body fat levels. People in this situation and those with a strong genetic component may be structurally and functionally different to the mildly overfat and in fat loss programs their outcomes may not be as favourable. They might need different programs to achieve similar levels of success as programs aimed at mildly fat people.

## THE ENERGY RESERVE FUNCTIONS OF FAT

Fat makes up between 15–30 per cent of total body mass in the average female and around 12–25 per cent in the average male.

**Table 3.1:** Body composition of young males and females of the same height and weight

|  | Females | Males |
|---|---|---|
| Height (m) | 1.65 | 1.65 |
| Weight (kg) | 57.0 | 57.0 |
| Total body water (kg) | 29.5 | 36.0 |
| Lean body weight (kg) | 41.0 | 50.0 |
| Fat (kg) | 16.0 | 7.0 |
| Fat/body weight (% fat) | 28.0 | 12.0 |

*Source:* Frisch (1994)[4]

Conversely, men have more lean body mass (mainly muscle) and more body water than women (see Table 3.1).

These proportions change with age, degree of muscularity, fitness levels and a range of other factors, but they generally represent the difference between the sexes. Each gram of fat is the equivalent of around 9 kcal of energy. Hence, a person with 15kg of body fat will have the equivalent of 135 000 kcal of potential energy. To put this in perspective, for a person who weighs 70kg, it requires about 100 kcal of energy to walk 1km. It also requires around 2000 kcal of energy to keep the average sized person alive for a day. This is called the resting metabolic rate (RMR). So theoretically, fat stores provide enough energy to keep the average person alive for around 60–70 days. For the average person to perform normal daily activity and to meet energy requirements of metabolism, a daily consumption of around 2000–2500 kcal of food is required.

---

1 kcal = 4.2 kilojoules

---

*Glucose* (a basic form of carbohydrate) is the other main source of energy used by the muscles. This is a more immediate source of fuel than fat in that it can be used in the absence of oxygen. An analogy would be the difference between using paper (glucose) and wood (fat) as fuels in a fire. Paper is quick to start, but also burns out quickly. Wood is slower to get going, but is a much more effective form of fuel over a longer period.

Glucose is present in the body in three main locations: liver, muscle and blood. In the blood it circulates as glucose and in the liver and muscle it is stored as glycogen, which is a series of glucose molecules joined together. Total storage volumes in each of these locations is shown in Table 3.2.

In contrast to fat, glycogen has to be stored with water. Each

**Table 3.2:  Total energy storage in a 70kg man**

|  | | Amount stored (g) | Energy (kcal) |
|---|---|---|---|
| 1. Glucose | | | |
| Blood | | 20 | 80 |
| Liver (as glycogen) | | 80 | 360 |
| Muscle (as glycogen) | | 350 | 1500 |
| | Total | 450 | 1940 |
| 2. Fat | Total | 15 000 | 130 000 approx. |

gram of glycogen is stored with about 3 grams of water, making it very bulky as an energy store.

As can be seen from Table 3.2, compared to the huge stores of fat in the body, only about 450g of glycogen is stored for energy use. As one gram of glycogen (carbohydrate) has an energy value of 4.5kcal, total stores amount to around 2000kcal, or equivalent to 1 day's energy supply. Although this storage capacity can be increased, and perhaps even doubled through various nutritional techniques such as *carbohydrate loading*, glucose stores can't be relied upon for long term survival in times of food shortages. Indeed, if we were to store as much glycogen as provides the equivalent energy of fat stores in the body, humans would need to be the size of elephants to accommodate the volume of glucose and water! Fat, therefore, is a very efficient and valuable store of energy.

## SUBCUTANEOUS AND INTRA-ABDOMINAL FAT STORES

Fat cells exist in all parts of the body with four exceptions: the eyelids, parts of the oesophagus, the brain and the penis. The main location of concern to the weight watcher is *subcutaneous fat*, which is stored below the lower surface (*dermis*) of the skin (see Figure 3.3). This gives skin its 'rounded' or cushioned feeling when pinched.

On some parts of the body subcutaneous fat is thicker, and fat cells more numerous, than on others. The abdomen, as we've seen, is a site of greater adipocyte size and numbers in men; the buttocks and gluteal region more so in women. Women also tend to store more fat around the triceps than men, and this area is harder to pinch using traditional skinfold measures, in some women. The female breasts are almost entirely composed of fat and connective tissue, the former serving as an extra energy reserve during pregnancy and lactation. The extra energy require-

**Figure 3.3: Location of subcutaneous fat**

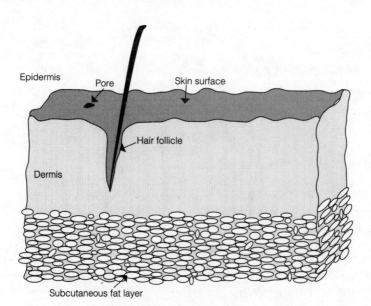

Epidermis

Pore

Skin surface

Hair follicle

Dermis

Subcutaneous fat layer

*Source:* Frisch, R., 1994, 'The right weight: Body fat, menarche and fertility', *Proceedings of the Nutrition Society*, 53:113–129.

ments of breast-feeding have been estimated at between 300—400 kcal per day.[3]

Harvard University's Dr Rose Frisch, who is an expert in female body composition and fat stores, claims that subcutaneous fat stores in the hips and buttocks, as well as the breasts, also help to augment food supplies during pregnancy. Says Frisch: 'The main function of the 16kg of stored female fat, which is equivalent to 600MJ [about 140 000 kcal], may be to provide energy for pregnancy and for about 3 months lactation'.[4] Intra-abdominal fat stores on the other hand may be less functional and may interfere with liver function leading to different disease risks.

## AN OVERVIEW OF FAT CELL FUNCTION

Figure 3.4 gives a general overview of the storage (*lipogenesis*) and breakdown (*lipolysis*) of fat into and out of fat cells. The mechanisms controlling lipolysis and lipogenesis are complex and elaborate and a detailed understanding of them is beyond the

**Figure 3.4:  Storage and breakdown of fat**

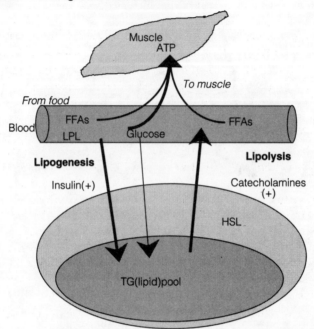

scope of this book. However, an overview of the fundamental processes involved follows.

Ignoring protein and alcohol, Figure 3.4 shows that fat is carried in the bloodstream in the form of free fatty acids (FFAs) which have been broken down from triglycerides (TGs) from food and fat stores. The other main source of energy is sugar (glucose). Glucose is used up readily in muscle tissue as energy when it is available in significant amounts, such as after a meal (hence the thick arrow from glucose to the muscle in Figure 3.4). Otherwise, the muscle uses FFAs as its main source of energy (such as after overnight fasting, in which case there would be a thick arrow from FFAs to the muscle in Figure 3.4). FFAs are efficiently stored as triglycerides in the fat cell. The obligatory biochemical cost of storage of fat as body fat is about 3 per cent of the energy available in the fat. The cost of converting glucose to fat on the other hand (*de novo lipogenesis*) is around 25 per cent of the available energy in the carbohydrate, which helps to explain why *de novo* lipogenesis is now not thought to occur significantly in humans under normal physiological conditions i.e. non-forced feeding of carbohydrate.[5,6]

## THE FATE OF FAT IN FOOD

Fatty acid molecules travel through the blood as either FFAs or as triglycerides (TGs) which is a group of three fatty acid chains joined by a glycerol molecule. An analogy may be footballers roaming the streets on their own, or joined by a team manager. Triglycerides cannot get directly into the fat cell because their molecules are too big, so the team needs to be broken down into FFAs and glycerol units like the footballers having to pass single file through the door into a nightclub. Once inside the nightclub (fat cell), they join up with the glycerol into a 'team' again and are stored as TGs.

Keeping the nightclub analogy, our footballers have to get past a doorman. In the fat cell, the main 'doorman' is the hormone *insulin*, which is formed in the pancreas and secreted into the bloodstream in response to a rise in blood sugars. Before a meal (low insulin), the doorman has the exit open allowing FFAs to leave to supply energy for the body. After a meal (high insulin), the doorman closes the exit and opens the entrance to allow FFAs to enter. Insulin also activates an enzyme, *lipoprotein lipase* (LPL) in the fat cell. This acts like a 'spruiker' outside the nightclub touting for business. Adipose lipoprotein lipase (ALPL) breaks FFAs off the TG so that they can enter the fat cell.

Insulin also acts as a doorman for the muscle cell but here the functions are somewhat different because he has two entrances to control. Before a meal he has the 'fat door' open to allow FFAs into the muscle cell to provide it with energy. He also activates muscle LPL which breaks down the TG teams passing by to allow FFAs to get through the door. After a meal, he closes the fat door and opens the 'glucose door' so the muscle switches from running on fat to running on glucose. (Interestingly, if the muscle needs a lot of energy such as during exercise, the glucose goes straight in through another door that insulin has no control over.)

The process of lipolysis is shown on the right hand side of Figure 3.4. Basically, when the body needs more energy than is currently available from food, triglycerides in the fat pool are broken down into FFAs plus glycerol and sent to the muscle via the bloodstream to help out. It's as if someone has run into our 'nightclub' and called all the footballers out to help out in another building down the road. The process is triggered by another enzyme which, like all enzymes, causes a reaction but doesn't take part in that reaction. *Hormone Sensitive Lipase* (HSL) is the enzyme involved in this removal of fats from the fat pool. It does so under orders from a range of chemical 'alarmists' in the bloodstream, particularly the *catecholamines*, or hormones secreted from the *adrenal glands* at the top of the kidneys. The catecholamines, therefore, facilitate lipolysis, but inhibit lipogenesis. Insulin, on the other hand, facilitates lipogenesis, but inhibits lipolysis.

## THE FAT CYCLE

The process of conversion of fatty acids in the blood stream to triglycerides in the fat cell and back again to fatty acids in the bloodstream is a constant one. The biochemical term for the rebuilding of FFAs into TG in the fat cell is *esterification.* There is an active cycle of free, or *unesterified,* fatty acid uptake into the fat cell which is then re-esterified within the fat cell. Hence there is an ongoing process of lipogenesis, lipolysis and release of FFAs.

Fats which are released into the bloodstream during lipolysis are liberated from their glycerol base and transported to the muscle via the blood to be used as fuel. However, more fat is usually released than is used up. At rest, it has been shown that about 70 per cent of fats released into the bloodstream are re-esterified back into the fat cell, but this decreases to about 25 per cent after the first 30 minutes of a low intensity exercise session. When the exercise is completed, some fats continue to be burned in the recovery process, but about 90 per cent of those released which have not been used up are then re-esterified, and stored back in the fat cell until another day. In exercise then, about one-half of the increase in fat oxidation contributing to the extra fuel supply comes from a reduction of the percentage of re-esterification (fats re-entering the fat cell), rather than an increase in fats being released from the fat cell.[7]

The process of re-esterification may be important for the fat loss process as some studies have shown that the degree of re-esterification, in contrast to the extra fat used up, may be influenced by the post- and pre-exercise meal of the exerciser. Injecting glucose into a fasted subject for example, has been shown to increase the re-esterification of fats back into the fat cell more quickly than it inhibits lipolysis, possibly due to the increase in insulin following a glucose load which then has an inhibitory effect on lipolysis.[8]

**Figure 3.5:  Lipogenesis**

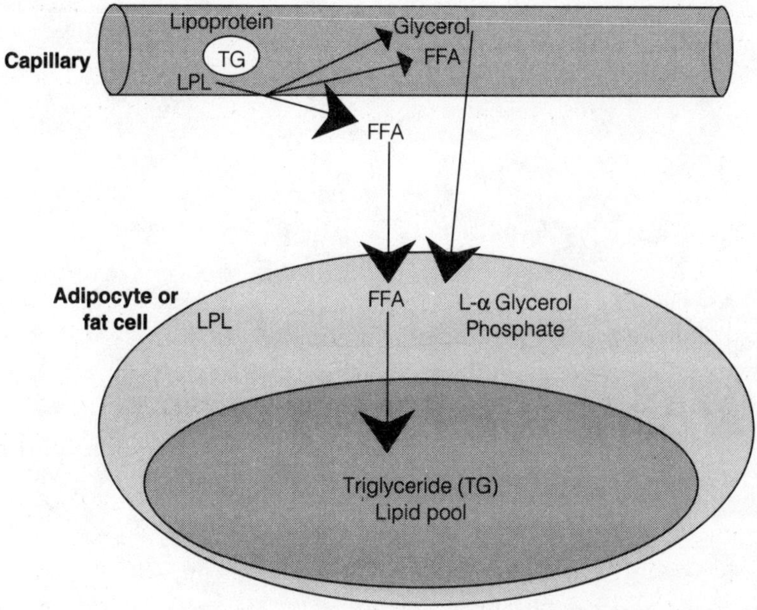

FAT STORES IN MUSCLE

As well as depot and circulating stores of fatty acids, muscles can call on a more immediate source of fat for energy if required. This is in the form of fat droplets in the muscle tissue itself. Because of its physical proximity, this is probably the first store of fat that is tapped by the muscles once energy demands call on extra fat to help out. It makes sense then that well-trained athletes are able to utilise this source of fat much earlier and more efficiently than the non-trained (probably because of a higher level of LPL in trained muscle and because fat is channelled to muscle in preference to the adipocyte because it is used on a more regular basis). This may also help to explain, along with muscle catabolism, why well-trained endurance athletes tend to be very thin in the muscles which are not being used in their event—the upper body muscles of the marathon runner for example.

Of course, all this is just a cursory glance at what happens in the fat cell and in the muscle tissue. The process is much more complicated and to start to make sense of this, we need to examine the processes of lipogenesis and lipolysis separately.

**Figure 3.6:** **Lipolysis**

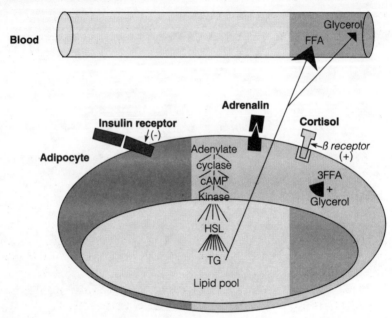

## Lipogenesis

The process of lipogenesis is shown diagrammatically in Figure 3.5.

As we have seen, circulating triglycerides (TGs) in the blood-stream are packaged in the blood into *lipoproteins* which are then split into free fatty acids (FFA) and glycerol by the enzyme LPL to get into the fat cell. Once inside the cell, the FFAs interact with glycerol which is derived from glucose, to form TGs again. These TGs are then stored in the fat cell's large lipid storage droplet. This whole process of esterification of fatty acids (and re-esterification of those released and not used up in the muscle) requires very little energy and assures that an abundant supply of FFA is

---

MYTH-INFORMATION

*Figure wrapping is claimed by some commercial organisations to reduce body fat because of 'secret' herbal mixes applied before wrapping. Physiologically these have no effect on lipolysis. Any weight loss effect in the short term is due to fluid losses alone.*

---

readily available as a metabolic fuel. The key factor of importance here is that it is predominantly fats in food, in the form of FFAs which make fats in the fat cell. As we'll see in Chapter 5, glucose, or sugar, is not converted to fat except under unusual circumstances.

## Lipolysis

The process of lipolysis, or breakdown of fats is summarised in Figure 3.6.

There are a range of *receptors* on the membrane, or surface of the fat cell, which respond in a number of different ways to a range of messenger chemicals, or *hormones*. These are a bit like locks and keys which open the cell up for a cascade of events which then result in the enzyme HSL being activated to break down TG into FFA plus glycerol for release into the bloodstream. This *metabolic cascade*, or amplification of chemical reactions, is common in nature and enables a much larger response to a small stimulus to occur. Enzymes, or catalysts, also take part in these reactions enabling them to be sped up to the rate necessary for a biological response.

There are over 30 different receptors, or 'locks' which have been identified to date on the fat cell membrane, and many more likely to be discovered. The β (beta) receptors are important receptors which facilitate lipolysis. The hormones which lock into the β receptors are adrenalin and noradrenalin (catecholamines), both of which are involved in responses to stress. Factors affecting catecholamine production (and therefore potentially lipolysis), include exercise, cold, stress, caffeine and some other stimulant drugs, such as the amphetamines (which have, in the past, been the basis for some weight control drugs).

The lypolytic hormones 'unlock' a cell receptor (Figure 3.6), and the signal is then amplified through proteins inside the cell which in turn generate a substance called *cyclic AMP* (cAMP) which continues a cascade of events ending in the activation of the enzyme *hormone sensitive lipase* (HSL). This is the final step in the enzymatic attack on stored triglycerides which are hydrolysed (broken down) into FFA and glycerol. The circulating FFAs released may then be re-esterified back into the fat cell, or released to the circulation or taken up by other tissues to produce energy. The final combustion of FFAs in cells to produce energy is known as *fat oxidation*, and is the process by which stored body fat is ultimately used.

### Factors influencing lipogenesis and lipolysis

Although fat moves continuously through the fat cycle, at times lipogenesis dominates and at other times lipolysis dominates. The overwhelming factor influencing the balance is the state of feeding, with fasting favouring lipolysis and feeding favouring lipogenesis, as already discussed. These directly correspond to the demand for fat as fuel.

Another condition which favours lipolysis is stress, either physical or psychological, such as exercise or a fearful situation. Adrenalin causes an increase in lipolysis with FFAs being released into the bloodstream *anticipating* a demand for fat as fuel. If the situation passes without the need to use the extra energy, such as with exercise, the fat returns from the fat cycle back to the fat cell. In other words, an increase in lipolysis does not always correspond to an increase in fat utilisation for energy.

A number of other factors can influence the balance of lipolysis and lipogenesis. A large fat mass tends to increase the amount of lipolysis and thus the amount of FFAs available for energy needs. Insulin, catecholamines, cortisol and sex hormone levels can also alter the balance. Fat cells in the hips, buttocks and breast are more responsive to female hormones than the fat cells on the abdomen, which are more prolific in men.

### IMPLICATIONS

1. Hyperplasia of fat cells is more likely during early adolescence and may be a danger time for future obesity.
2. Fats in the diet are converted into body fat (lipogenesis) whereas body fat from other sources of energy such as glucose (de novo lipogenesis) is negligible.
3. Fat, from both fat cells and intra-muscular sources, is utilised more readily by trained athletes than the untrained, hence physical activity at all levels is likely to be more lipolytic in the trained.
4. Breast-feeding enhances energy use significantly and therefore should benefit the long term body fat levels of the mother, as well as being important for the health of the baby.
5. Eating immediately after exercise might decrease post-exercise

fat oxidation. Therefore recommendations for athletes to replace glycogen stores after strenuous exercise need to be separated from advice to overfat people doing physical activity to lose fat where immediate replenishment may not be optimal.

6. Stressors in the form of physical activity, cold and caffeine may increase catecholamine production and aid in the break-down of stored body fat.

# 4

# Bioenergetics and metabolism

SUMMARY OF MAIN POINTS

- Bioenergetics is the study of energetic events occurring in living organisms; it covers energy (food) intake and energy expenditure.
- Fat is the most energy dense nutrient, containing more than twice the energy of carbohydrate or protein.
- Energy expenditure is made up of resting metabolic rate, the thermic effect of food and the energy cost of physical activity.
- Bigger people have a higher metabolic rate mainly because of a greater resting metabolic rate from a higher fat-free mass.
- Even very small females require an energy intake of around 1200kcal per day to maintain energy balance.

The living cells of the human body are in a constant state of molecular activity, where they are used, degraded and synthesised to maintain life. These actions require *energy* which is defined as '*the capacity to perform work*'. This definition does not, however, describe the many biological functions that either require or liberate energy in the body.

Understanding what energy is and how the body acquires, converts, stores, and utilises it is the key to understanding how humans can perform activities. It also provides the basis for understanding how fat is used as an energy source, or *substrate*, and how this may be optimised for best maintenance of body fat levels. The study of energetic events occurring in living organisms, which commenced in the 18th century, is called *bioenergetics*.

## BIOENERGETICS

Energy can take a number of forms:

- nuclear
- light
- chemical
- electrical
- mechanical
- thermal
- magnetic
- potential

According to the laws of thermodynamics, all forms of energy are interchangeable and energy is neither gained nor lost, it merely changes form. With respect to humans this means that the body cannot create or destroy energy, but it can convert one form of energy to another. Humans use chemical energy from food for synthesis and other metabolic processes. The chemical energy from food is converted to various forms such as mechanical energy which results in movement, chemical energy to make hormones, or electrical energy to conduct nerve impulses. Unless energy is stored in the body, it is eventually lost, mainly as heat (*thermogenesis*). Since living organisms are governed by the laws of thermodynamics, an energy balance equation has been used to forecast changes in body mass when changes in energy intake or expenditure occur, although this is not as clear cut as was once thought (see Chapter 7).

## ENERGY CURRENCY

Energy in the biological cycle originates from the sun. Plants convert solar energy to chemical energy through a process called *photosynthesis*. Humans then eat plants and/or animals which also eat plants. From these we obtain the calorie/containing components or *macronutrients* known as carbohydrates, proteins, fats and alcohol, which contain stored energy. These are then broken down by the body's cells to provide energy. The processes of

**Figure 4.1:** **The processes of energy formation and storage from the macronutrients carbohydrate, protein and fat**

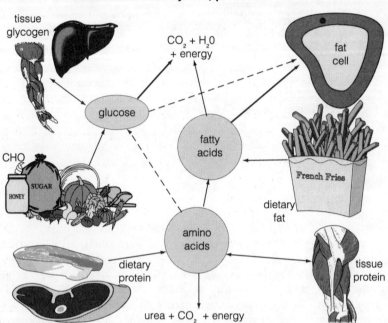

energy formation from the different types of food (carbohydrate, protein, fats) are shown in Figure 4.1. The thickness of the arrows in Figure 4.1 also illustrates the ease with which each nutrient is converted to energy or stored as fat in fat cells, a thicker arrow indicating easier conversion.

The body's cells trap the chemical energy released from food in a high-energy compound known as *adenosine triphosphate* (ATP) which is stored in small quantities in every cell. When energy is needed (say to transport glucose into the cell), the ATP gets broken down to adenosine diphosphate (ADP), thereby releasing the energy needed for the cell's processes.

Energy derived from fat, carbohydrate, a protein and alcohol is used in the body for *catabolic* processes which are involved in the break down of cell tissue and for *anabolic* processes which build up cell tissue. If protein is called upon to fuel these processes, the basic protein units (*amino acids*) are first converted to glucose through a process called *gluconeogenesis*. In addition to supplying the energy for these processes, the four nutrients, but especially protein, can also be the building blocks for growth, such as when muscle size increases with exercise. The sum total of energetic events which occur in the body, i.e. *anabolism* plus *catabolism*, is known as *metabolism*.

$$Metabolism = anabolism + catabolism$$

To provide the energy for these events, the body has three major reserve energy stores; glucose which is stored in the liver and muscle as glycogen, protein which is stored primarily in muscle, and fat, the majority of which is stored as *depot* fat, subcutaneously, around the internal organs and intramuscularly.

Eventually all energy is reduced to heat, therefore the energy produced by living organisms is measured in terms of heat production as kilocalories (kcal). One kilocalorie is defined as the amount of heat energy required to raise 1 kilogram of water 1° Celsius (C) at 15°C. The energy values of food are measured in a similar way through *direct calorimetry* where a food item is placed in a chamber called a 'bomb calorimeter' and combusted in a vat of water. Using the conversion formula above, the rise in water temperature is recorded as kilocalories. The four basic food components have the approximate energy values per gram shown in Table 4.1.

Given the energy values shown in Table 4.1, it is important to understand the abbreviations of terms as these are often confused in the popular press. What the lay person usually refers to as '1 calorie' is actually '1000 calories', or '1 kilocalorie'. One real calorie is actually a very small unit, and hence it is multiplied by 1000 to give a kilocalorie (or kcal). This is sometimes also referred to as 1 Calorie (spelt with a capital C). New metric measures also confuse the issue with 1 cal being equivalent to

**Table 4.1: Energy value of macronutrients**

| | |
|---|---|
| Carbohydrate (1g) | 4.5 kcal (19kJ) |
| Protein (1g) | 4.5 kcal (19kJ) |
| Fat (1g) | 9 kcal (38kJ) |
| Alcohol (1g) | 7 kcal (29kJ) |

**Table 4.2: Notation of energy measurement units**

| Basic unit | Abbreviation | Conversion |
|---|---|---|
| calorie | cal | 4.2J |
| Joule | J | 0.238 cal |
| *Usual unit* | *Abbreviation* | *Conversion* |
| kilocalorie* | 1kcal (1000cal) | 4.2kJ |
| kilojoule | 1 kJ (1000J) | 0.238kcal |
| megajoule | 1MJ (1000kJ) | 238kcal |

*Note:* generally referred to as a calorie in the popular media

4.184 joules, or 1 kcal being equal to 4.184 kilojoules (notation 'kJ'). To round off the figures, 1 kcal is generally regarded as being equal to 4.2 kJ. Table 4.2 shows the notations and conversion factors from calories to joules.

## PRODUCTION OF ADENOSINE TRIPHOSPHATE FROM FOOD SOURCES

Now we have outlined the source, storage depots and measurements of energy, the next step is to examine the production of the energy rich molecule adenosine triphosphate (ATP), the energy currency of the body. This is made up of adenosine with three phosphate groups attached (Figure 4.2). ATP is found in every cell. It is the common pathway for energy production for driving bodily functions. At the microscopic muscle filament level, the reduction of ATP to adenosine diphosphate (ADP) is the energy source used for contraction. That is, energy liberated from the reduction of ATP to ADP allows the basic protein filaments of muscle, actin and myosin, to slide across each other to cause muscular contraction.

Energy is derived through the cleaving-off of high energy phosphate bonds from the ATP molecule to form ADP+P (see Figure 4.2).

The energy for the re-synthesis of ATP from ADP+P comes from nutrients as they get broken down in their catabolic pathways or from the small energy reserves in muscle called the creatine phosphate system. The direct breakdown of nutrients only occurs by itself at very high temperatures. However, in the human body it must occur at normal body temperature (36.5 to 37.5°C), and this is done through a series of stepped chemical reactions, which are catalysed by many different enzymes. Enzymes are proteins that have the ability to promote specific chemical reactions without the need for high temperatures and without being changed or degraded themselves in the process. They can therefore be used over and over again.

### MYTH-INFORMATION
*Corset-like 'sweat pants' sold to reduce fat around the buttocks have only the superficial effect of 'tightening' bulges. They cannot and do not reduce body fat.*

**Figure 4.2:  The creation of ATP for energy**

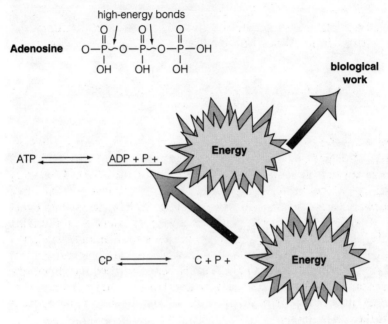

## METHODS FOR MEASURING ENERGY EXPENDITURE

The energy content of foods, or the energy requirements of physical activities, can be measured in a number of ways.[1] Basically there are three categories of measures that are used:

### 1. DIRECT CALORIMETRY

Direct calorimetry can also be used to measure energy expenditure in the form of heat loss from the human body. This requires placing a person in a small chamber in which all the heat released is measured. Unfortunately, such chambers are very expensive and are only present in well-established research laboratories. Direct calorimetry can also be used to measure the energy content of food through 'bomb calorimetry', as previously discussed.

### 2. INDIRECT CALORIMETRY

This calculates energy use directly from measurements of the amount of oxygen ($O_2$) consumed, carbon dioxide ($CO_2$) and nitrogen produced (the latter to eliminate protein metabolism in

**Figure 4.3:  Inside a standard metabolic chamber**

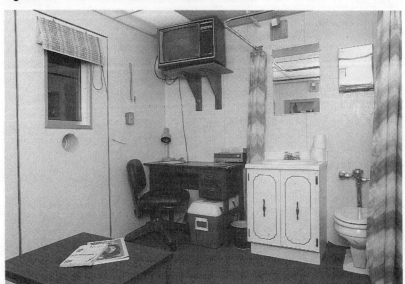

the equation). This can also be done in a chamber (metabolic or respiratory chamber) over periods of 24 hours or more, or it can be done with a hood system over a period of minutes or hours. An example of a metabolic chamber is shown in Figure 4.3. From indirect calorimetry equations, the amount of each type of energy substrate being used can also be calculated. This is expressed as the respiratory exchange ratio (RER), or respiratory quotient (RQ).

The RER, which is based on the ratio of oxygen ($O_2$) consumed to carbon dioxide ($CO_2$) produced, can provide information about whether the predominant energy source being used is carbohydrate or fat. The theory behind this is that more oxygen is required to burn fat relative to the amount of carbon dioxide produced. In fact, the ratio of $O_2$ to $CO_2$ is around 0.7 when fat is the total fuel being oxidised. On the other hand, when carbohydrate is used as a fuel, equal amounts of $O_2$ and $CO_2$ are involved. Where carbohydrate is the sole fuel therefore the ratio of $O_2$ to $CO_2$ is 1.0.

At rest, the terms respiratory exchange ratio (RER) and respiratory quotient (RQ) can be used interchangeably, although strictly speaking there is a difference. RER refers to the exchange ratio of gases expired, whereas RQ is a measure of the ratio of fuel use at the tissue level. RER, which is more relevant for our purposes here, is derived from the chemical calculations shown in Table 4.3.

**Table 4.3: Formula for respiratory exchange ratio (RER)**

The respiratory exchange ratio (RER) = $\dot{V}CO_2$ / $\dot{V}O_2$
Fast energy production requires FAST FUEL or glucose from carbohydrate

| $C_6H_{12}O_6$ | + | $6O_2$ | = | $6CO_2$ | + | $6H_2O$ |
|---|---|---|---|---|---|---|
| carbohydrate | | oxygen | | carbon dioxide | | water |

The RER (ratio of carbon dioxide produced to oxygen consumed) for oxidising (burning) glucose is 6/6 or 1.0.

Long slow energy production requires fat

| $C_{57}H_{104}O_6$ | | $80CO_2$ | = | $57CO_2$ | | $52H_2O$ |
|---|---|---|---|---|---|---|
| triglyceride (fat) | + | oxygen | | carbon dioxide | + | water |

The RER for most fats is around 0.7 (i.e. here it is 57/80 = 0.713)

As seen in Table 4.3, an RER of 1.0 indicates carbohydrate is the energy substrate being used, 0.71 means that only fat is being used. When a mixture of 50/50 fat and carbohydrate is being used the RER is 0.86 and 0.82 is a usual figure for energy use in a fasting state.

## Doubly labelled water

A more recent technique for energy expenditure measurement, which is likely to become more common in the future, is the *doubly labelled water* technique. This was first used with humans in the early 1980s and involves loading a person with water which has been labelled with two stable isotopes, deuterium and a form of oxygen, and then measuring the differential elimination of these from the body through the urine. From this information, scientists can calculate the rate of use of oxygen and production of carbon dioxide over the period measured to a high degree of accuracy. The method is simple, safe and non-intrusive. At present its main limitation is the expense of the labelled water and the mass spectrometer needed to analyse the output.

## 3. NON-CALORIMETRIC METHODS

These measure energy intake or output by a variety of methods including food and physical activity diaries and questionnaires. All these methods are based on a number of assumptions and many are only very rough estimates of energy expenditure. Methods based on heart rate diaries are also not very accurate.

As can be seen from Figure 4.4, body weight is the most

important component of total energy expenditure, mainly because of the association between resting metabolic rate and fat free mass (FFM). Because bigger people have more total body mass and therefore also FFM, total energy expenditure will be greater. On the other hand, even the lightest female measured at rest in a metabolic chamber over a 24-hour period will expend at least 1200kcals, suggesting that a minimum dietary intake of 1200kcals is necessary for normal daily functioning.

## COMPONENTS OF ENERGY EXPENDITURE

When dealing with the area of managing body fat levels we must have a basic understanding of how energy is balanced in the body. We consume on average anywhere from 1500kcal–2500kcal per day. This adds up to an energy intake of about 555 000–1 million kcal (2.33–4.17 kJ) per year. But what about expenditure? How does the body balance energy intake with expenditure? Why can some individuals seemingly consume relatively greater quantities of food than others, and at the same time end up with lower stores of body fat? Dr Klaas Westerterp and his group from the University of Limberg in the Netherlands, have estimated that over the course of a lifetime, there is an actual discrepancy between energy intake and energy expenditure of only around 1 per cent, making the system an extremely well balanced one.[2] What this implies, of course, is that body weight is not just equal to the amount of energy intake minus energy expenditure, but that energy intake + expenditure must change, as a function of a number of factors, to help balance the system. To understand this, we need to understand the components of energy expenditure. Components of total energy expenditure in an individual are shown in Figure 4.5.

Figure 4.5 shows that there are three main components of energy expenditure.

1. Resting metabolic rate (RMR) or basal metabolic rate (BMR), which equals sleeping metabolic rate (SMR) and arousal.
2. The thermogenic effect of food.
3. Exercise, or daily physical activity and spontaneous physical activity (SPA).

The vast majority (i.e. around 70 per cent) of daily energy expenditure (EE) in the average person is accounted for by RMR. Thermogenesis contributes about 15 per cent and daily physical

**Figure 4.4:    24-hour energy expenditure as a function of body weight**

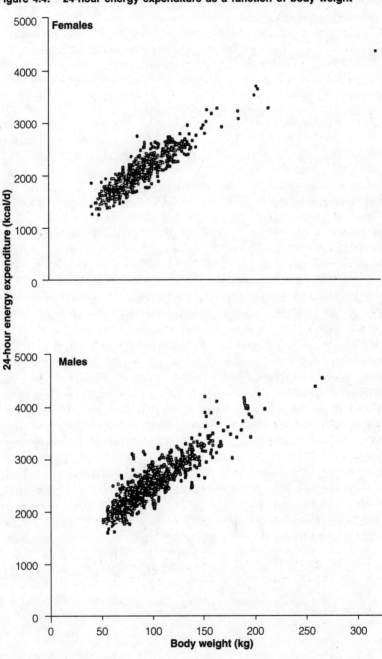

activity is the most variable being around 10–25 per cent in sedentary individuals.

## 1. Resting Metabolic Rate (RMR)

The term *metabolism* describes the sum total of the thousands of dynamic chemical reactions that occur in the body to sustain life. RMR is the sum total of energy needed to keep the body going at rest. It can be likened to an idling engine. The synthesis of new tissue, for example, during growth and pregnancy have significant metabolic cost. Body size is also related—a bigger person has a generally higher metabolic rate. To extend the analogy of the idling engine, this would be a truck that is required to carry a heavier load. To do this might require a bigger engine which would then burn more fuel while idling. Resting metabolic rate (RMR) can be estimated from equations based on height and weight. One common formula for doing this is shown in Table 4.4.

There are two basic factors which determine metabolic rate (MR) at any given moment: the number and size of respiring cells, and the metabolic intensity of those cells as determined by the work being done and how efficiently energy transformation occurs to meet the body's demands. Resting metabolic rate (RMR) is the energy required to sustain life while an individual is at rest, but still awake. Basal metabolic rate (BMR) is often used synonymously with RMR and the energy required to sustain life at the lowest level, which is during sleep, is called the sleeping metabolic rate (SMR). The main determinants of metabolic rate are fat-free mass (FFM), fat mass (FM), age and sex. A 'determinant' is a factor which explains differences in metabolic rate between individuals.

RMR accounts for 60–70 per cent of daily energy expenditure. Excess consumption of energy or overfeeding causes an increase in RMR, while underfeeding, such as very-low-calorie diets (VLCDs) and fasting result in a decreased RMR. Most of these changes are due to changes in fat-free mass (FFM) and the thermic effect of food (which is dependent on the calorie load). There may also

**Table 4.4: Formulae for estimating resting metabolic rate (RMR)**

Males

RMR = 66 + (6.22 × wt (lb)) + (12.7 × ht(in)) − (6.8 × age)

Females

RMR = 655 + (4.36 × wt (lb)) + (4.32 × ht(in)) − (4.7 × age)

**Figure 4.5: Components of total energy expenditure**

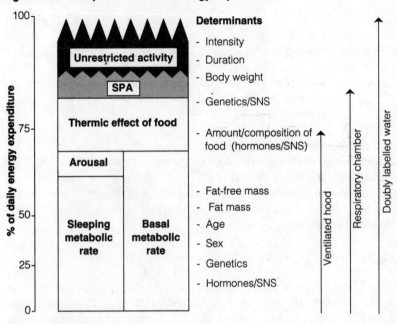

*Source:* Ravussin & Swinburn (1993)[3]

*Notes:* SPA = Spontaneous physical activity
SNS = Sympathetic nervous system activity

be some 'adaptive' changes which result in a metabolic rate (MR) which is greater (for overfeeding), or less (for underfeeding) than predicted.

## Factors thought to modify the metabolic rate

### Fat-free mass

The amount of FFM (which includes all non-fat components such as muscle, organs, bones, blood) is by far the biggest determinant of MR. The higher the FFM, the higher the RMR and total MR. Obese people have higher FFM (mainly muscle) in order to carry around their extra weight. Thus, they also have a higher MR compared to lean people. Skeletal muscle metabolism accounts for approximately 50 per cent of RMR and about 75 per cent of MR when active during exercise. At a given body weight, an individual with a greater proportion of FFM to fat mass (FM) would have a higher metabolic rate.

## Fat mass

As body fat levels increase so does RMR. Most of this is due to the increased FFM, but even at the same amounts of FFM, the person with the higher fat mass (FM) has a higher RMR. Similarly, as FM decreases, RMR will decrease and tend to 'brake' the reduction in body fat which might otherwise occur.

## Age

Recent research estimates that RMR decreases at a rate of approximately 2 per cent per decade between the ages of 20 and 70 years. This reduction is accounted for primarily by decreases in FFM which is mostly due to reduced overall physical activity. However, at the same levels of FFM and FM, older people have a slightly lower RMR.

## Gender

For a given body weight, females have a lower RMR than males due to a lower FFM to FM ratio. Females also have a slightly lower RMR than males independently of FFM, FM and age, most probably due to the effects of sex hormones on RMR. Several studies have shown that energy expenditure varies within the female menstrual cycle. During the pre-ovulatory (*progesterone*) stage, RMR appears to be 6–15 per cent lower than during the pre-menstrual (*oestrogen*) stage. RMR may also be reduced in women taking progesterone-only oral contraceptives.

## Genetics

FFM, FM, sex and age account for about 70–80 per cent of the differences in RMR between people. Other genetic factors account for some of the remaining differences. This suggests that RMR is at least partially genetically determined. These findings are supported by studies involving identical (*monozygotic*) and non-identical (*dizygotic*) twins which showed that identical twins are more alike with respect to RMR than non-identical twins.

## Sympathetic nervous system (SNS) activity

The SNS is that part of the nervous system involved in generally speeding up the body's responses, for example through increased heart rate, constriction of blood vessels and release of hormones such as adrenalin. The SNS also stimulates lipolysis resulting in the release of free fatty acids (FFA). The degree of SNS activity may have a small influence on RMR.

*Ambient environmental temperature*

When the environmental temperature is low, maintenance of normal body temperature at 37ºC is an active process requiring extra energy. For this reason more energy needs to be expended in cold conditions than in warm. The cooling process (for example, sweating) is more energy efficient than the heating process (for example, shivering). The use of a sauna bath may result in fluid loss (and therefore weight loss), but not significant *fat,* or energy loss. Similarly, exercising while rugged up to increase sweating is only likely to have a short term effect on fluid loss and no extra effect on fat loss over and above the exercise. On the other hand exercising in the cool or cold, while only lightly dressed, would require that the body increase its energy use to maintain body temperature. Of course, this needs to be balanced by the injury protection benefits of warming up muscles before exercising.

*Physical activity*

One question which is often asked is whether physical activity has a carry-over effect on RMR? In the short term immediately after exercise, there is an excess post-exercise oxygen consumption (EPOC) which reflects an ongoing excess metabolic rate. The duration of EPOC is dependent on the duration and intensity of the exercise, but it may last for a few hours. In the longer term, the question of whether fit people have a higher RMR after the EPOC has disappeared (say 24 hours after an exercise bout), is less clear. A recent review of all the major work carried out in this area[3] suggests that regular physical activity does have a positive effect on increasing RMR but this is mainly because of the relative increase in FFM in the body. The longer term benefit of regular exercise on metabolism is probably more related to changes in the respiratory exchange ratio (RER) than RMR.

## 2. Thermogenic responses

Thermogenesis describes increases in the MR above RMR in response to things such as food intake, exposure to cold or heat and the body's physiological responses to fear or stress.

### Thermic effect of food

The thermic effect of food (TEF), also called diet-induced thermo-genesis, represents increases in MR above RMR resulting from the energy costs of digestion, absorption, transport, metabolism and storage of food consumed. Consumption of food produces a transient increase in MR until it is assimilated. When these processes are complete, MR returns to the pre-meal state. The TEF is the major form of thermogenesis, accounting for approximately 10–15 per cent of daily energy expenditure. Many studies have been done to examine if obesity is related to a decrease in TEF. In a recent review of all these studies it was discovered that several found a difference between the lean and obese and several found no difference. It is important to remember that even in those studies which found a difference, it was only of the order of about 1 per cent of energy expenditure.[4]

The major factors which influence the TEF are the meal size and composition. A higher TEF is seen with a higher calorie load and a higher proportion of protein. The energy cost of processing protein is very high (~ 20% of its calories) compared to fat and carbohydrate which only cost a few per cent of its calories. Other factors which affect TEF are palatability of the food and time of the meal, as well as a person's age, genetic factors, physical fitness and some specific foods.

> MYTH-INFORMATION
>
> *'Food combining' to control body weight has no foundation in fact. The body is very capable of combining foods (like meat and vegetables). If it wasn't, humans would have evolved a completely different physiology.*

*Caffeine:* Several studies have shown an increase in MR of up to 10–30 per cent for 1–3 hours after administering oral or intravenous caffeine.[5] It appears that the optimal amount is the equivalent of about 2–3 cups of instant coffee per day. Caffeine use in athletes has also been shown to increase performance by increasing lipolysis and, therefore, sparing carbohydrate during endurance events.[6] However, recent work also suggests that the effect of caffeine is not as great in the obese as in normal weight individuals.[7]

*Spicy foods:* Spicy foods such as chillies and curries, which contain an ingredient known as capsaicin, have been shown to elicit small increases in TEF.[8] The use of spices not only adds flavour to low-fat dishes therefore, but also may have a small, transient effect on increasing MR.

*The importance of TEF*

Most researchers do not regard TEF as a major cause of obesity. According to Ravussin and Swinburn:

> . . . one can safely state that individual differences in the thermic effect of food can only account for small differences in daily energy expenditure. This implies that a minimal weight gain will increase energy expenditure (mostly in relationship to resting metabolic rate and the energy cost of physical activity) and will therefore be sufficient to offset any impairment in the thermic effect of food.[9]

### 3. Energy cost of physical activity

This is simply the energy expended above RMR that is needed to produce movement. The energy cost of physical activity can account for significant energy expenditure in very active people. However, in overfat, unfit individuals it typically represents between 15–30 per cent of total energy expenditure.[10] There are different ways of categorising movement, but one helpful way when looking at whole populations is to divide it into occupational, recreational and incidental physical activity (PA). Occupational activity, which is the PA required to perform a person's job, has been declining for decades as automation and energy-saving machines continue to increase. Recreational activity is that chosen by a person to do in his or her leisure time, such as walking, playing tennis, or cycling. People have considerable control over such planned activities and it seems they are on the increase. However, even in an active person this still only amounts to a few hours per week which is a small proportion of the week's energy cost of PA. Incidental PA is essentially all the rest of the movement and is the activity needed to carry out daily activities. It includes stationary activity such as gesticulations, fidgetting and arm movements, as well as walking around the house, getting in and out of cars, walking around the shops and so on. There is no information about changes in incidental activities, but it seems highly likely that energy-saving devices, convenience parking, push-button remote controls, ergonomic designs and hundreds of other small influences add up to a sizeable decrease in incidental PA over the last decade. Small daily increases in energy expenditure, whether through planned exercise or through 'incidental activity', might have a significant effect on long term fat losses. Small, gentle increases, rather than large sudden increases in energy use are less likely to create an adaptive response by the body and are hence more likely to have a positive effect over the long term. Chapters 12 and 13 look at ways of increasing fat loss through physical activity.

## IMPLICATIONS

1. Obese people have a higher fat mass and fat-free mass than lean people.
2. Obese people generally need a higher energy intake to maintain weight than lean people.
3. Lack of weight loss on a diet of <1200 kcal is generally due to under-reporting of food intake.
4. Significant fat loss is invariably accompanied by decreases in FFM and thus decreases in RMR. This will tend to reduce the rate of weight loss. Exercise during weight loss helps to preserve FFM and prevent some of the decrease in RMR.
5. A reduction in fat in the diet will result in a greater decrease in energy intake than a similar (gram for gram) reduction in other nutrients.
6. Substrate utilisation (i.e. nutrient use as energy) can be measured through the respiratory exchange ratio (RER), using the ratio of inhaled to expired air, and the means of measuring RER are becoming more and more portable.
7. Physical activity expends energy both during and after the activity. RMR appears to remain elevated after activity. However, the level and duration of increases are a function of exercise intensity, duration and frequency.
8. Wrapping and 'sweating it off' will lose water, but not fat. Remember that maintenance of body heat in cold conditions is an active process requiring energy.
9. It is reasonable to use spices that increase RMR—particularly those high in the ingredient capsaicin—to add flavour to low-fat dishes.
10. Caffeine in moderation may be a possible aid to fat loss but at worst, is not likely to interfere in the fat loss process. Denial therefore is not a necessary pre-requisite for fat loss.

11. Caffeine and spicy foods may have small effects on metabolic rate, but the major opportunity for increasing metabolic rate still must be through increases in physical activity and reductions in fat in the diet.
12. Increasing incidental physical activity should be used as well as increasing planned exercise.

# 5

# The role of fat in energy balance

SUMMARY OF MAIN POINTS

- *De novo* lipogenesis is the term used for making fat from other nutrients such as carbohydrate and alcohol.
- *De novo* lipogenesis is not thought to have a significant role in humans under normal physiological (day-to-day living) conditions.
- Unlike carbohydrate and protein, fat is not finely balanced in the body.
- Fat (from the diet and adipose tissue) is the energy buffer for the body—it makes up the difference between what the body obtains from non-fat calories and what it needs.
- Alcohol is the highest priority fuel for burning, but unlike protein and carbohydrate, it does not reduce hunger.
- Energy balance and fat balance are essentially equivalent.

In the traditional teaching of energy balance, it has been assumed that, in humans, there is a relatively free conversion of non-fat calories to fat calories for storage. This is no longer so; now fat nutrients are thought to be more fattening than nutrients gained from either carbohydrate or protein.

The reasons that fat was thought to be a major contributor to obesity were twofold: its high energy density of 9 kcal/g, and its relatively inexpensive conversion to fat storage (about 3–5 per cent of its energy) compared to carbohydrate at 4 kcal/g and about 25 per cent of its energy needed to convert it into fat for storage. A better understanding of the physiology of macronutrient (carbohydrate, protein, fat, alcohol) balance has now added a more powerful reason: macronutrients are largely handled separately by the body and, under modern living conditions, dietary fat is essentially the only macronutrient which ends up in fat stores. Indeed, obesity can be seen as the 'price' paid for eating a high-fat diet and burning little fat through exercise since it is the gain in fat mass and fat-free mass which brings the body back into energy and fat balance.[1]

Physiologically, therefore, all calories are not equal and fulfil quite different roles in energy balance. The role of fat is to provide energy reserves and fat in the diet has little impact on the active maintenance of energy balance through appetite mechanisms or stimulating fat burning. But does this mean that fat calories are more important in the cause or treatment of obesity? Changing diet composition while maintaining the same total calories does not result in weight changes over the long term, and increasing the calorie intake, irrespective of its composition, does cause some weight gain in the long term. However, we don't live in a calorie controlled environment. Under conditions of ad libitum (free) eating, where foods are selected from a wide variety of choices and eating is at liberty in generally unrestricted amounts, the composition of the diet does have a substantial and important effect.

Increasing the dietary fat content results in a slow fat gain in all but the very active and decreasing the dietary fat content results in slow fat loss in people who are overfat. Therefore, the quality of the diet (i.e. fat:carbohydrate ratio) affects the quantity of the diet (i.e. the total calories). In the development of obesity, high fat content and high total calories are both important because they occur together, but the critical insight is that fat is, to a large extent, responsible for total calories anyway.

## THE ENERGY BALANCE PARADOX

An anecdotal survey of people living in the modern world reveals an interesting paradox in energy balance. On the one hand, it seems that the body has an excellent, in-built energy balancing system which for some people keeps them at the same body mass, or at least within a variance of about 1 per cent, over decades.[2] This is a remarkable feat if one considers that over a

10-year period the body can balance about 10 million kcal in, with 10 million kcal out, without the individual having to consciously count a single one! On the other hand, for some people, this system seems to go very wrong as they gain fat over time, despite their best conscious efforts not to. Has the system broken down in these people? This seems unlikely and the probable resolution of the apparent paradox is that the body has excellent balancing mechanisms for all types of calories except one—fat. So high-fat diets and low fat burning can result in fat gain without the usual energy balancing systems detecting it, because they are not designed to detect it.

ENERGY BALANCE

The energy balance equation has underpinned most efforts to explain the energy dynamics of obesity. Obesity is characterised by high energy stores and usually a high energy intake and expenditure (metabolic rate). To reach a state of obesity, there needs to be a chronic imbalance between energy intake and expenditure over a long period of time. However, as we have seen in the previous chapter, an initial positive energy balance will cause energy stores to increase (both fat mass and fat-free mass) which in turn causes an increase in energy expenditure, due mainly to the increased resting metabolic rate from the greater fat-free mass. At some point, the weight gain and increased energy expenditure will offset the original imbalance and a new equilibrium will be achieved.

Therefore, the energy balance equation helps to explain *how* a positive energy balance leads to weight gain and how a new steady state is achieved. However, it fails to answer two critical questions: *why* did the positive energy balance occur in the first place and *why* does it remain chronic over long periods? The answers to these questions may come from an understanding of the regulation of individual macronutrients (carbohydrate, protein, fat, and alcohol). However, separating out each macronutrient balance equation can only be valid if the biochemical highways *do not* allow a free flow of nutrients. What are the restrictions for converting one nutrient to another for storage and, in particular, are glucose and alcohol converted into fat through the process called *de novo* lipogenesis?

## *DE NOVO* LIPOGENESIS

The lipogenic enzymes needed to make new fat are present in humans but in far smaller concentrations than in other animals. The rate of *de novo* lipogenesis in the liver can be estimated in normal humans and has been uniformly found in the order of only a few grams per day. In other words, even on a high-carbohydrate, low-fat diet, the body would not be expected to turn more than a few grams of the excess carbohydrate into fat.

While the liver may synthesise a small amount of fat from non-fat precursors, other tissues, such as skeletal muscle, may simultaneously be burning fat for fuel. Therefore, *net whole body* fat synthesis will only be present if the former is greater than the latter, which is rarely the case. Examples of conditions which result in net lipogenesis are forced overfeeding of carbohydrate (i.e. up to 5000kcal of carbohydrate per day in the resting state), some disease states such as cirrhosis or HIV infection, states of malnutrition, direct infusions of simple sugars intravenously (such as during intravenous nutrition) or into the abdominal cavity (such as during peritoneal dialysis). These can swamp the body's ability to use glucose as an energy fuel or store it as glycogen, and under these conditions, some of the glucose is forced to convert into fat. However, this state is very difficult to achieve by eating or drinking the carbohydrate, even in the form of simple sugars.

In 1988, Dr Kevin Acheson and his colleagues from the University of Lausanne in Switzerland showed that drinking 2000kcal of simple sugar solution (500g of dextrin maltose) resulted in only a few grams of fat production, and even massive carbohydrate overfeeding (about 5000kcal/day, 85 per cent carbohydrate) for several days after saturation of glycogen stores resulted in about 150g/day of new fat production.[3] Since that time, these results have been replicated through a number of different studies.[4]

---

MYTH-INFORMATION

*Contrary to popular opinion, carbohydrate-rich foods are not as fattening as those high in fat. This is not only because carbohydrates (sugars) contain less energy, and require more energy for storage, but because carbohydrate is not converted to fat in humans under normal physiological conditions.*

---

Clearly, net *de novo* lipogenesis requires forced overfeeding of carbohydrate and does not occur under the conditions of ad libitum (at liberty or free) eating in normal individuals. Excessive consumption of carbohydrate (to the level of 50 per cent more than normal), has been shown to lead to increased fat deposition if maintained over the long term (14 days or more), but the indications are that this is because of fat sparing through increased carbohydrate use as an energy substrate, rather than conversion of excess carbohydrate to fat.[5]

## MACRONUTRIENT BALANCE

There is some inter-conversion between nutrients such as protein being converted to glucose (gluconeogenesis) for release into the bloodstream, but under normal conditions, the capacity to convert one nutrient into another *for storage* is very limited. Also, humans have little capacity to 'waste' extra energy by burning it off. This process, which has been termed *luxuskonsumption*, is common in animals such as rats but is very limited in humans. Therefore, the examination of each macronutrient as a separate entity is necessary and is summarised below and in Table 5.1.

### Alcohol

There is an inconsistent relationship between reported alcohol intake and body mass index, with many studies showing that drinkers of large amounts of alcohol have lower body weights.[6] This has led to hypotheses that alcohol calories may be subject to inefficient oxidation, thereby diminishing the impact of alcohol calories on energy balance. In heavy drinkers, there does seem to be an inefficient burning of alcohol because the addition of alcohol to a weight maintenance energy diet does not result in weight gain.[7,8] Virtually all ingested alcohol is metabolised in the liver and this process produces energy. None of it is converted directly into fat. The main pathway is via the enzyme *alcohol dehydrogenase* and this should theoretically produce 7kcal/g of alcohol. However, alcohol also appears to induce another series of liver enzymes to burn it and this pathway produces far less energy for use than the usual one.

Alcohol, perhaps because of its toxic potential, is the top priority fuel for burning and, if present, displaces fat and, to a lesser extent, carbohydrate and protein as fuel sources for energy

**Table 5.1: Effect of increasing macronutrient intake on energy balance**

| Increased intake of: | Non-fat oxidation | Fat oxidation | Fat storage | Appetite | Weight gain |
|---|---|---|---|---|---|
| Carbohydrate | ↑ | ↓ | ↑ | ↓↓ | – |
| Protein | ↑ | ↓ | ↑ | ↓↓ | – |
| Alcohol | ↑ | ↓ | ↑ | ?↑ | ↑ |
| Fat | – | – | ↑↑ | ? | ↑↑↑ |

*Notes:* Oxidation is the burning of fuels for energy, the total amount of which is determined by the demands of the body. Non-fat oxidation refers to the sum of carbohydrate, protein, and alcohol energy being used.

needs. Hence, while alcohol does not directly turn into body fat, it will certainly send any spare fat in the diet into storage. So it appears that the so-called 'beer gut' may not be full of beer calories, but rather full of the chips and nuts that accompanied the beer which have been sent to the fat cells for storage. A sobering fact though is that although alcohol does stimulate its own burning, it does not satisfy hunger, and indeed may stimulate appetite. The nature of beer is such that the type of food that is likely to be eaten with it will probably be high in fat (can you imagine beer and fruit rather than beer and nuts?). The sugar which is in the beer, wine and mixes may have an effect on reducing appetite and therefore counter the stimulation of appetite by the alcohol. Overall, we could consider alcohol as 'half-balanced' as a form of energy in the body and a potential promoter of weight gain.

## Protein

Protein stores are mainly in muscle and their size is dependent on need. In other words, muscle mass increases in response to growth stimuli such as certain hormones, physical training and weight gain, but not in response to more protein in the diet. Eating more steak and eggs will not produce bigger biceps, just more protein for use as energy. Protein is a minor source of fuel for the body, usually supplying less than 20 per cent of total energy needs. Any protein not needed for replacement of the structural proteins (e.g. muscle) and functional proteins (e.g. enzymes and some hormones) is used for energy. Protein, along with carbohydrate, is a second priority fuel for burning. It does satisfy appetite (in fact, it is the most potent satiating nutrient) and can be considered 'fully balanced', (i.e. the amount taken in is usually balanced by the amount used up) and therefore protein is an unlikely cause of weight gain.

## Carbohydrate

Carbohydrate stores (glycogen) are very small and tightly controlled in the body. Only relatively small increases in glycogen storage capacity can be gained, for example by the carbohydrate loading techniques employed by endurance athletes, which may increase stores by up to 2.5 times the normal amounts. Carbohydrate calories from the diet keep this small storage space topped up but are mainly used for current energy needs and displace fat as an energy source. Carbohydrate is, therefore, a second priority fuel for energy use, after alcohol. Unlike alcohol and fat, carbohydrate and protein are the main regulators of appetite by satisfying hunger and producing satiety. While the exact mechanisms for this are not known, parts of the complex cascade of responses are being discovered and they appear to involve stretch nerve fibres in the stomach, hormones released from the gut, increases and decreases of certain nutrients in the blood, and a whole series of neurochemical responses in the brain. The final target for appetite control is in the hypothalamus in the brain. Carbohydrate, like protein therefore, is 'fully balanced' by influencing both its own burning and satiety mechanisms.

MYTH-INFORMATION

*'Fat metabolisers', which are generally forms of amino acids, are often claimed to 'convert fat to body fuel'. However, scientific assessment shows they are substances which are easily synthesised by the body and have no effect on body fat.*

## Fat

Fat is handled very differently by the body compared to the other nutrients. Body fat stores are large and not actively controlled and fat intake has no influence on its own use as a fuel (oxidation) and very little influence on appetite. Fat (from the diet or adipose tissue) is the energy buffer for the body in that it makes up the difference between what the body obtains from non-fat calories and what it needs to keep functioning. It is the last priority as a fuel. Fat is therefore not balanced at all and in a sense the body is 'blind' to fat, both in the diet and in the fat stores when it comes to balancing up its energy needs. Excess fat is therefore the most powerful dietary promoter of weight gain.

Energy balance and fat balance are essentially equivalent. This means that on a day when a person has eaten 200kcal more than they have burned, about 200kcal of dietary fat will be stored as body fat. If a person is 200kcal under, the body will pull about 200kcal of fat out of the fat stores to make up the deficit.

Table 5.1 shows how carbohydrate and protein intakes are fully balanced or regulated (suppress appetite and promote their own oxidation), alcohol intake is only half balanced (promotes its own oxidation only), and fat is not balanced at all. As originally proposed by Professor J-P. Flatt from the University of Massachusetts, a high-fat diet therefore tends to lead to a passive over-consumption of calories which may become chronic because of the weak or absent metabolic controls on fat balance.[9]

All this implies that a reduction of fat in the diet is all that is required for reducing body fat. There are certain advantages and disadvantages of this approach, as opposed to the old notion of calorie counting. Some of these are shown in Table 5.2. Reducing fat, for example, doesn't feel like 'dieting' and is therefore much easier than total food restriction. However, there is a perception that a low-carbohydrate diet is more effective because much of the weight lost is fluid which occurs relatively quickly. In a low-fat diet, the loss is slower but is more likely to come from fat than fluids. The low-fat approach also allows large volumes of food to be eaten with a minimum of restrictions, hence not resulting in the problems of hunger which occur with normal 'diets'. In general, this whole approach leads us away from the traditional notion of *calorie counting* to one of ad libitum low-fat eating—a much more practical and effective approach to fat loss

**Table 5.2:** The reduced-fat, ad libitum approach to weight loss: advantages and disadvantages

| Advantages | Disadvantages |
| --- | --- |
| Doesn't feel like 'dieting'. | Weight loss slower than expectations. |
| Simple to understand and follow. | Difficult for some 'dieters' to adjust to. |
| Large variety of food choices. | Not enough low-fat options available. |
| Large volumes of food. | High-fat foods seen as most pleasurable. |
| No problems with hunger. | Requires monitoring of fat intake. |
| Not anti-social. | Some food and meal planning needed. |
| No calorie counting. | Diet of the general population is high in fat. |

and one which is considered in much more detail in Chapters 8–11.

## IMPLICATIONS

1. Reducing dietary fat in favour of carbohydrate and protein is likely to be the most effective long term dietary fat loss technique.
2. Alcohol denial may not be necessary on a fat loss program, but restriction of dietary fat is advisable if maintaining alcohol intake.
3. Because alcohol in the body is only partially balanced, control of hunger may be more of a problem with alcohol consumption in terms of fat gain than the alcohol itself.
4. Carbohydrate intake in the presence of a low-fat diet can be surprisingly high, thus allowing for greater satiation and less hunger.
5. The use of a low-fat ad libitum eating plan, in contrast to reduced total calories may result in a less immediate *weight* loss, but a slower and more permanent reduction in body *fat*.
6. A low-fat eating plan is likely to be a much more liveable option for most people than trying to get them to eat less total food.

# III
# MEASUREMENT

# 6

# Measurement and assessment of fatness

## SUMMARY OF MAIN POINTS

- Accurate measurements of body fat, mass and distribution require a variety of techniques and there is no one entirely satisfactory measure.
- A combination of measures is usually necessary to determine health risk.
- Validity, reliability and sensitivity of measures are an important indication of their worth.
- BMI is a good measure of body mass; waist circumference of fat distribution; skinfolds are useful measurements in the hands of experienced operators and with the non severely obese.
- New measures of central fat, such as abdominal diameter, may have important uses in the future.

Typically, the most commonly used measure of body fatness has been body weight. This is then compared with a table of 'ideal weights' prepared by life insurance companies on the basis of actuarial data, relating weight to the risk of an early death or to average weights in the population, and some measure of over-weight calculated on the basis of population figures.

The advantage of weight is that it is a simple, accurate and reliable measurement. For individuals, significant changes in weight over the long term usually reflect significant changes in body composition. However, weight is often not a true reflection of obesity—particularly in those in the population (e.g. athletic males) who might have high body density due to muscular structure—nor a good indication of health risk, because measures of weight (in contrast to body fat distribution) do not correlate highly with illness risk. Height is, of course, a confounding factor and hence the calculation of body mass index, or BMI, which corrects for height, has become the norm.

More recently, it has been realised that BMI is also not always a good representation of fatness, again because of the bias against those with a high body density (i.e. those with a high fat free mass to fat mass ratio, FFM:FM). Hence there has been a recent move towards new measures of total body fat and fat distribution, including the better use of simple anthropometric measures such as height, weight and circumference measures. There has also been a move to develop cost-effective machines which accurately measure fat, in contrast to body mass.

## ACCURACY OF MEASURES

The accuracy of any measure of body fatness, as with other physical and psychological tests, can be gauged in at least three ways; by its *validity, reliability* and *sensitivity.* Each of these are scored on a scale from 0 to 1.0, where 0 implies a low degree of accuracy and 1.0 a perfect measure.

*Validity* refers to the degree to which a measurement actually measures what it purports to. Without validity, any technique is useless.

*Reliability* refers to the degree to which the measurement used measures the same on different occasions.

*Sensitivity* refers to the degree to which the measurement instrument can detect subtle changes, and derive different scores as small changes occur.

Given these three factors, measures of fatness can then be rated for their usefulness in the practical situation. We have divided these into (a) manual measures, (b) machine measures of fatness, and (c) measures of body fat distribution.

## THE CONCEPT OF 'IDEAL WEIGHT'

Over the years, several attempts have been made to establish a series of 'ideal weight' measures as a goal for people to aim for. One of the first of these, the 'Broce Index', was estimated in kilograms by taking 100 away from height (in cm). In other words, a person 180cm tall might be expected to have an 'ideal weight' of 180–100=80kg. Ideal weights for height have also been developed over the years (beginning in the late 19th century in the US) based on actuarial, or death statistics. More recently, ideal measures of body mass index, skinfolds and fat distribution have been used (see below). However, scientists have yet to agree on a measure of 'ideal', and now generally accept that a variety of the measures discussed below have to be combined.[1]

### Manual measures of body mass and fat mass

*Weight*

Weight is a measure of the force of gravity acting as the total mass of an object. As such it reflects not only the overall size of the body but also the density of the combination of body tissues, including bone, muscle and body organs. Fat is lighter than water and therefore adipose tissue is lighter than muscle and organ tissue (which are mainly water) and both are lighter than bone. Increases in *weight* might therefore mean an increase in fat mass, muscle mass and/or fluid (remember, glycogen is stored with three times its weight in fluid). Over the long term, it's true that changes in weight generally reflect changes in body fat, but in the short term the use of scales is not recommended as a measure of success of a fat loss program. Weight scales also vary significantly, from a sensitive bar balance or high quality electronic scale to the less sensitive but more often used bathroom-type scales.

The validity of weight as a measure of body fatness then is only fair, especially in certain types of individuals such as mesomorphic (muscular) males and elite athletes. Reliability of the measure on the other hand is quite high. Sensitivity is also reasonably high (i.e. around 0.8) detecting small changes in body mass. But, of course, this is not sensitive to *fat* as distinct from changes in other body tissue. Weight, therefore, is limited as a measure of fatness, except where combined with some other measures.

> ### MYTH-INFORMATION
> *Weight loss through heat treatments such as saunas and steam baths represents fluid losses through sweat. These techniques have no permanent effect on fat loss.*

### Body Mass Index (BMI)

BMI (sometimes also called 'Quetelet's index') was developed to account for the influence of height on body mass. The measure is weight (in kg) divided by height (in m) squared, i.e. BMI = wt(kg)/ht(m)$^2$. Recommended ideal range for BMI is 20–25 kg/m$^2$. Overweight is regarded as over these upper levels and the different levels of obesity are defined as shown in Table 1.2 in Chapter 1.

BMI has as its main advantage the ability to be used in large scale population studies. It requires only two measures; height and weight, which can both be measured accurately by a person with minimal training. It suffers similar deficiencies to weight in that it is less valid in those with a mesomorphic build, and particularly athletic men. The validity of BMI, although higher than weight, is lower than is necessary for a good measure of body fatness. Validity has also been found to be higher in women than men and to be significantly influenced by body build.

Comparisons with other anthropometric measures, at least in large populations, show the usefulness of BMI measures. Its reliability is relatively high, but as with weight, this can be influenced by fluid content. Sensitivity could be expected to be similar to that for weight as height is not expected to change significantly, except with age. The BMI therefore is useful for large scale population studies and, in combination with other measures, is useful for individuals. Some researchers have called for the total abandonment of BMI. However, according to Lohman. '. . . BMI needs to be included with skinfolds or bioelectric impedence and other laboratory body composition measures of muscle, bone, and fat'.[2]

The limitations of BMI, as with weight, need to be understood in working with individuals, i.e. there is a need to apply other assessments (including a practised 'calibrated eyeball technique') to raw BMI data.

### Skinfold thickness

Skinfold thickness has traditionally been used to measure body

**Figure 6.1:  Fat and muscle content influences on body mass index (BMI)**

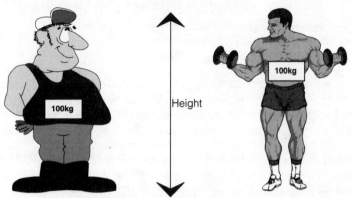

**Normal ranges are
20-25 for females and males**

Height

100kg

100kg

**Weight (kilograms) / Height (metres)²**

fatness in athletes. The original validation studies in general populations were carried out using under-water weighing, or cadavers, as the 'gold standard' measure and there have been traditionally two main equations; that developed by Jackson and Pollock in 1981[3] using 3, 4 or 7 sites, and that developed by Durnin and Womersley in 1974[4] using 4 sites. Measurements from these have then been extrapolated, perhaps unwisely, to estimate body fat percentage in normal populations.

Skinfold thickness is measured by the use of special calipers at certain sites on the body to measure the thickness of subcutaneous body fat. Calipers to measure skinfold thickness can range from a $10 plastic type to a $300 version and have been found to give different outcomes. Skinfold measurements are also extremely dependent on the experience of the measurer. Studies carried out comparing the effectiveness of measurers show that the variability even between experienced measurers can be anything up to 20 per cent.

Skinfolds appear to be reasonably useful measures of body fat in capable hands for adults between 10–40 per cent body fat, but may under-estimate fat in those over 40 per cent fat. Recently, extrapolation of skinfold thickness to percentage of body fat has largely been dropped in favour of just using the sum of skinfolds. This means that skinfolds are not necessarily an indication of percentage body fat, but the sum of skinfolds can give indications of relative changes in body fatness. In 1988 a conference on the standardisation of measurements was conducted in the US and from this a standardisation manual is now available[5] giving 47 different anthopometric dimensions. For detailed reference on how to take these measures, this manual should be consulted. The main sites generally used are:

*Biceps:* Bicep skinfold is measured as the thickness of a vertical fold raised on the front part of the arm, midway along a vertical line joining the upper shoulder and the elbow joint.

*Triceps:* Tricep skinfold is measured in the midline at the back of the arm between the lateral projection of the shoulder and the elbow joint. The skinfold is measured with the arm hanging loosely and comfortably at the subject's side.

*Subscapular:* This is picked on a diagonal level at approximately 45 degrees to the horizontal in the natural cleavage of the skin parallel to the lower scapular border. To find the site, the measurer can feel for the scapula, running the fingers around the border until the lower angle is identified. Another method is to bend the subject's arm behind his or her back such that the scapula stands out. Apply the calipers 1cm away from the pinch raised by the finger and thumb.

*Suprailiac:* The suprailiac skinfold is measured in a line immediately above the iliac crest or upper hip, on the right hand side of the body. A fold of fat is grasped just above the hip in a midline along the body turned side-on. The fold taken should follow the natural cleavage of the skin at about a 45 degree angle.

*Abdominal:* Abdominal measurement should be done approximately 3cm lateral to the midpoint of the umbilicus (navel) and 1cm below this. A horizontal skinfold should be raised with the left hand and its thickness measured to the nearest 0.1cm.

*Thigh:* Thigh skinfold is located at the midline of the front of the thigh, mid-way between the crease at the hip and the top of the patella, or kneecap. The subject should flex the hip to assist location of the hip, or inguinal crease. The skinfold is selected while the subject is standing but shifting the body weight to the other leg. Calipers should be about 1cm lower than the finger pinch of the skinfold.

### The value of skinfold measurements

Skinfolds represent a relatively simple method of measuring general fatness and fat distribution. The validity of skinfold measures in the hands of an experienced measurer in people who are not

**Figure 6.2: Common skinfold sites**

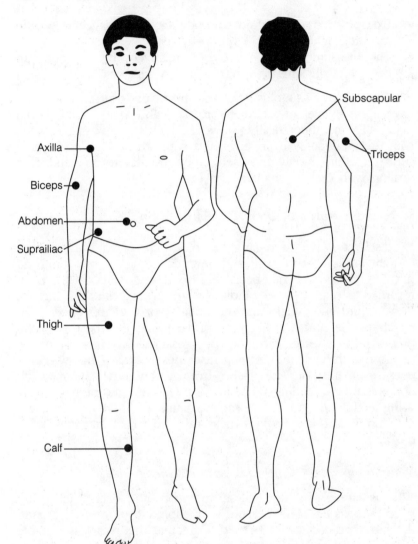

excessively obese can be quite high, however reliability is quite variable, depending on the measurer, and sensitivity quite low. Skinfold measures may be useful for elite athletes, or for testing small amounts of fat losses after a significant amount of fat has been lost. They have little value, though, for the very overfat or obese mainly because:

- It is difficult to get accurate measures on extremely large folds of fat.
- Extrapolation of skinfold to body fat percentage have little meaning at the higher levels of measurement.
- The measurement of skinfolds is relatively invasive and can be potentially embarrassing for a very fat person.

The value of skinfolds as a measure of body fat in those who have a high level of fat, therefore, is highly questionable, both practically and theoretically. However, they do have some value with the moderately overweight and with athletes (at least where sums of skinfold only are used), they are not recommended in dealing with overfat or obese subjects.

## Manual measures of body fat distribution

Fat distribution is now regarded as of equal or greater importance to total fat as a health risk and new techniques of measuring fat distribution have recently been developed. Abdominal fat has been regarded as one of the key indicators and measures of this include waist-to-hip ratio (WHR) and the Conicity or C-Index. Visceral fat, which in the future is likely to prove to be the most powerful predictor of disease, can only be measured *in vivo*, or in live organisms, through the imaging machines discussed below. However, estimates can be made from techniques that measure abdominal fat including WHR, and the C-index, and more recently using techniques to measure sagittal diameter (SAD), or a measure of abdominal thickness known as the abdominal diameter index (ADI).

### Waist-to-hip ratio (WHR) and waist circumference

WHR is a ratio of abdominal subcutaneous and visceral fat to hip subcutaneous fat.[6] The measure is 'anchored' to a measure around the hips because it had been thought that this was less variable to change. Recently though, Canadian researchers at Laval University in Quebec have suggested that waist measures alone may be

**Table 6.1: Risk levels for WHR and waist circumference**

| | Men | | Women | |
|---|---|---|---|---|
| Measure | Possible risk | Definite risk | Possible risk | Definite risk |
| WHR | 0.9 | 1.0 | 0.8 | 0.9 |
| Waist | 95cm | 100cm | 85cm | 90cm |

sufficient.[7] WHRs (or other ratio measures used, such as waist-to-thigh ratio) generally have a cut-off point determined by epidemiological studies with large populations. Figures of 0.9 for men and 0.8 for women are often used as the cut-off points for WHR beyond which increased disease risk is indicated, but in some studies the figures of 1.0 and 0.9 respectively are used (see Table 6.1).

Some research has shown that with fat loss in some people, there is a loss from the hips as well as the waist and therefore WHR can remain relatively constant. For this reason it is probably best used as an absolute measure of risk in the first instance of measurement, rather than a relative measure of change, and is best used in combination with other measures such as BMI.

Attempts are currently being made to incorporate WHR and BMI into a single formula, but so far these have not added to the individual predictive value of either single measure. Waist measurements suggested by the Laval group as indicative of disease risk are above 100cm for men and 90cm for women—irrespective of height. Researchers at Glasgow University[8] have compared waist measurements with BMI and have come up with the following conclusions for health promotion:

- men with a waist size of >102cm and women with a waist size of >92cm should be encouraged to lose weight
- men with a waist of between 94–102cm and women with a waist of 80–88cm should be encouraged not to put on any more weight
- men with a waist size of <92cm and women with a waist size of <80cm do not need weight management.

These figures have been rounded for ease of remembering and equate with those in Table 6.1.

WHR has a relatively high validity in the measurement of abdominal fat distribution, particularly in men and post-menopausal women, however validity may be affected by changes in hip size that occur with changes in body fatness. Reliability and sensitivity of waist measures alone is quite high, particularly in the hands of an experienced measurer.

Correct sites for measurement of waist and hips can vary and although there are currently attempts to standardise these, there is still controversy about the correct locations. There is general agreement that hips should be measured at the widest part of the buttocks as determined from side-on. Protocols for waist measurement include measures at umbilicus (the navel), which has the particular advantage of being easy to find, but the disadvantage of being almost at hip level in some obese women. Another waist site is mid-way between the lowest rib and the top of the iliac crest (hip bone), which has the advantage of bony landmarks but does not always capture the large abdominal mass in very obese people. In lean people the waist is the narrowest part between the chest and the hips but in obese people it can be the widest, therefore this is not recommended as a definition. Each has its disadvantages, but provided the measure is used constantly, the actual site becomes less relevant.

WHR and waist circumference measures have the advantages of being quick, non-intrusive and useful for large scale population surveys. WHR has disadvantages in making comparisons between varying groups of people such as is often seen in different cultural groups. Asian women, for example, have small hips and WHR measures are much less valid as an indicator of health risk. Negroid women on the other hand have large hips and buttocks and their health risk may be misinterpreted from WHR measures. Overall WHR, or waist alone, may provide a quick and simple indication of health risk. Waist alone can then be used to examine the success of a fat loss program in those groups where abdominal fat is stored readily.

### Skinfold measures

Skinfold calipers, discussed above, can be used as a measure of fat distribution as well as a total fat measure with specific body sites (such as subscapular) being used for relative measures of fat loss.

### Conicity Index (C-Index)

The C-Index was developed by Dr Radolfo Valdez and colleagues from Pennsylvania State University[9] in an attempt to combine the best aspects of BMI with WHR or body fat distribution. The C-Index quantifies fat shapes as lying between two extremes; the first a cyclinder, i.e. very lean, and the second, bi-conical (see Figure 6.3)

So far the C-Index has had only limited validatory research carried out on it, some suggesting it may not add significantly to other anthropometric measures. However, variations to this in the future may offer promise for a more sensitive measure.

The C-Index requires measures of height, weight and waist circumference and the following formula:

C = abdominal girth (at umbilicus) in metres/0.109/weight (kg)/height(m)

The range of scores is from 1.00 to 1.73 but, as yet, there are no normative figures for comparison. People scoring towards the low end, i.e. 1.00, are closer to the ideal than those scoring towards the high end, i.e. 1.73. The validity of the measure is so far unknown, although reliability and sensitivity could be expected to be quite high.

## Sagittal diameter (SAD) and abdominal diameter index (ADI)

Abdominal fat distribution is reflected in an extended abdomen or 'pot belly'. This consists of expanded subcutaneous fat cells as well as increased visceral fat. Its extent could, therefore, presumably be measured through a measure of sagittal diameter, i.e. the width of the waist from back to front. This has recently been investigated and a device developed for determining the measure

**Figure 6.3:** Cylinder and cone shapes which form the extreme measurements of the C-Index

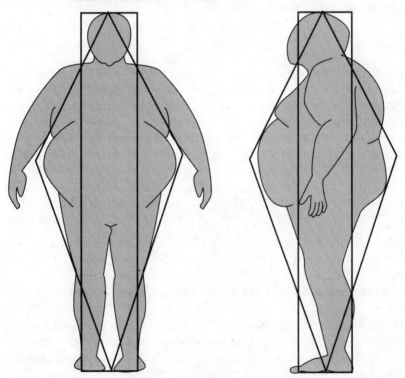

**Figure 6.4:   Kahn sagittal diameter calipers**

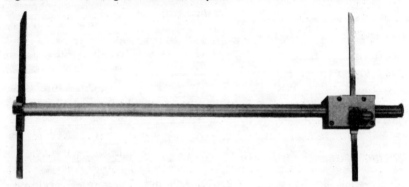

by Dr Henry Kahn from the University of Georgia. The device, called a sagittal diameter scale, measures the thickness of the abdomen at the umbilicus in either the lying or standing position (see Figure 6.4).

The higher the SAD measure, the greater the risk of disease, and although norms have yet to be established for this measure, indications from the Georgia laboratory suggest that a SAD measure of greater than 25cm indicates an elevated health risk.

The abdominal diameter index, also developed by the Kahn team, is an attempt to compensate for the lack of perfect predictability of the SAD measure of visceral fatness.[10] Because the sagittal measure includes not just visceral fat but bone, muscle and subcutaneous fat, the Georgia team have attempted to adjust for the non-visceral tissues that are incorporated in the SAD measure by dividing waist thickness by the girth of the mid-thigh. This also adjusts for overall body size as thigh thickness can be a good indication of total body size. ADI then becomes almost twice as powerful for the prediction of cardiovascular risk as the SAD alone.

Again there are, as yet, no well established norms for ADI. Early indications are that ADI measurements of over 0.5 (i.e. the cross-sectional thickness of the waist is over half the circumference of the mid-thigh) are highly predictive of risk for coronary heart disease.

## Machine measures of fat mass and fat distribution

Technological developments in the area have led to a number of different machines now being available for directly or indirectly measuring body fatness. Some of these are extremely expensive and would not be used in the normal day-to-day counselling situation. Others are now becoming more portable and more accessible and provide at least an opportunity for adding to other measures. The current range of machines include:

## Underwater weighing

Underwater, hydrostatic weighing, or *densiometry* as it is sometimes called, has been the 'gold standard' of fat measurement for many years. This is carried out by immersing the subject totally in water and corrrecting for air trapped in the lungs. The person's weight in air and their weight underwater are then calculated to determine body density, body volume and body fat percentage. The fatter a person is, the heavier he or she weighs in air and the lighter he or she weighs in water. Because it requires a lot of equipment and delicate measuring techniques, underwater weighing is generally reserved for research purposes or for measuring body fat changes in elite athletes. Validity is high, as is the reliability and sensitivity of the measure. The impracticality of this measure, however, limits it to research and teaching facilities, with little prospect for use in the practical counselling situation.

## Bio-impedance analysis (BIA)

BIA, which measures body fatness through electrical conductivity of body tissue, was introduced in the 1980s. A tiny imperceptible current travels through the water compartment of the body, which is proportional to the fat-free mass (FFM), there being very little water in fat. The more FFM, the more current is conducted. The impedance (or resistance to electical flow) is then put into an equation in the BIA machine to calculate the percentage of body fat. BIA machines are now small and portable and usually involve the wiring of electrodes onto the limbs of the body. The electrical current is slight and nothing is felt by the person being tested.

New developments have now led to BIA measures being combined with ordinary weight scales. By standing on the scales an undetectable electric current is passed through the soles of the feet and a measure of body fat is computed along with body weight. The combination of the two provides an increased diagnostic potential. A good deal of research has been carried out with BIA and comparisons with other measures such as near infrared analysis (NIR, see below) and other criterion measures. Indications are that BIA is significantly affected by fluid content

**Figure 6.5: A modern BIA weighing and body fat measurement device**

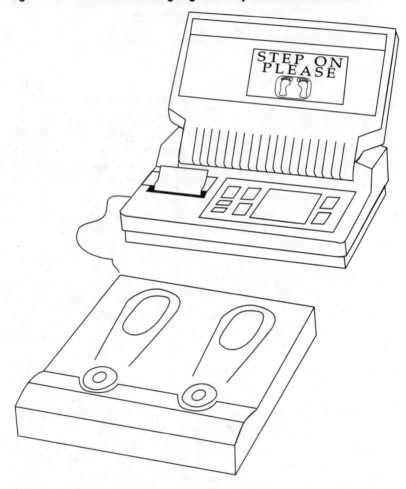

*Source:* Courtesy Wedderburn Scales, Tanita Corporation

of the body, and although reasonably valid, has a low reliability if not measured under similar conditions on each occasion.

*Near infrared analysis (NIR)*

NIR is a technique developed for the US Food, Drug and Agriculture Department (FDA) to measure fat content of beef carcases. It is based on the principles of light absorption and reflection using near infrared spectroscopy.

A small, hand-held probe, which emits electro-magnetic radiation through a central bundle of optic fibres is placed on the

**Figure 6.6:  NIR measurement**

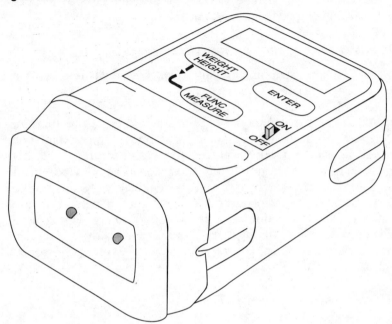

*Source:*   Courtesy Futrex–1000

skin at a selected site (usually the biceps for overall fat measurement). Optic fibres on the edge of the same probe absorb the
energy reflected back from the tissues and this is then passed on
to a spectrometer for measurement. Because muscle tissue is
denser than fat, muscle and fat can be determined by the end of
the light spectrum reflected back to the machine through several
centimetres of tissue. When multiple sites are used, the measure
is quite valid. NIR machines using only one site, (i.e. the biceps)
are now commercially available and reasonably portable (there is
even one hand-held device) and within the cost range of someone
working in counselling. They require one simple measure which
takes about 20 seconds, plus some other information fed into the
computer on age, sex, fitness level etc. The whole measurement
process takes only 1–2 minutes.

Again, the estimation of body fat is based on algorithms built
into the computer and hence the estimates are only as good as
the algorithms that support them. In general NIR has been found
to be slightly less valid than BIA measures, but reliability is unclear.
The sensitivity of the measure is unknown. Used by a skilful
operator it can be an effective motivational tool and can be used

to measure relative changes in body fat in different body locations, i.e. total and regional fat assessment.

### Dual energy X-ray absorptiometry (DEXA)

In 1987 the first commercially available dual energy X-ray absorptiometer (DEXA) was designed to measure the bone mineral content of the skeleton, especially at the spine, hips and wrist because they are common sites for osteoporosis. The machines, however, can accurately measure three body components (bone, fat and lean body tissue) both regionally and for the whole body and are now common in most hospitals. The method enables measurement of total fat as well as regional body composition. They use a very low dose of X-ray and scan a person in 20–40 minutes. DEXA is taking over from underwater weighing as the validation standard in fat measurement and body fat research, largely because of its accuracy, comparative ease of use, and widespread availability.

### Computerised tomography (CT) scans

Computerised tomography is another radiography technique of body fat assessment which has limitations because of its relatively high level of radiation exposure and cost. In the past, this has been used for assessing other forms of body tissue such as tumours, but it is also possible to assess body fat. The expense of the procedure, however, is unlikely to make it readily available. Also CT scans only do regional assessments rather than a total body fat record.

### Magnetic resonance imaging (MRI)

MRI is a technique based on the manipulation of protons and electrons in body atoms to give colour pictures of different body tissue. MRI machines are used for medical diagnosis such as the detection of cancers and, as such, are usually based in hospitals and are extremely costly. The future use of CT and MRI for more accurate measurements of abdominal fat is likely, but still only in a research context.

## REVIEWING THE MEASUREMENTS

As should be obvious from this cursory observation, there is no perfect measure of body fatness, or body fat distribution. The

**Table 6.2:  A summary of simple body mass and fat distribution measures**

| Measure | Advantages | Disadvantages | Indications |
|---|---|---|---|
| **Manual measures** | | | |
| Weight | • simple<br>• non invasive<br>• cheap<br>• reliable | • height not accounted for<br>• doesn't measure fat<br>• less reliable in the muscular | • population surveys<br>• individual tracking |
| Body mass index (BMI) | • as above<br>• includes height | • as above, except height included<br>• no fat distribution measure | • population surveys<br>• combined with other measure(s) |
| Skinfold thickness | • reasonably accurate<br>• total fat and fat distribution | • intrusive<br>• dependent on accuracy of tester<br>• limited for obese | • elite athletes<br>• lean to moderately obese individuals |
| Waist-to-hip ratio (WHR) and waist circumference | • distribution measure<br>• simple<br>• non invasive<br>• cheap | • less valid for women<br>• less valid in some ethnic groups<br>• less valid in those with small hips | • population surveys<br>• measuring risk<br>• combined with mass measures |
| Conicity (C-Index) | • adds height to fat distribution measure<br>• simple<br>• non invasive<br>• cheap | • calculation problems<br>• lack of uniform norms for risk | • as a check on WHR |
| Sagittal diameter (SAD) and abdominal diameter index (ADI) | • simple<br>• may be good measure of risk | • insensitive to change<br>• lack of norms<br>• cost | • as a check on WHR; C-index<br>• simple health risk measure |
| **Practical machine measures** | | | |
| Bio-impedance analysis (BIA) | • reasonably valid<br>• simplicity in recent models<br>• non invasive<br>• quick | • influenced by body hydration<br>• expense (around $A2000)<br>• different calculations needed for different ethnic groups | • clinical use<br>• combined with other measures |
| Near infrared analysis (NIR) | • reasonably reliable<br>• simple<br>• non invasive<br>• quick | • ? valid at extreme obesity<br>• local measure only<br>• expense ($A500-$1000) | • clinical use<br>• combined with other measures<br>• measure changes at various sites |

more easily usable measures discussed here are summarised in Table 6.2. Each has its advantages and disadvantages and these need to be considered carefully according to the situation. Some measures, e.g. BMI, WHR and ADI, might be combined in the practical situation and others would be left to more technical research procedures. Accessible new machine measures have improved the level of sophistication of measurement, but the degree of imperfection which remains in all current measures suggests there is an art to body fat measurement that is still required to accompany the science.

## IMPLICATIONS

1. All measures used should be appropriate to the individual and their situation, taking due concern for the privacy and sensitivity concerns of the individual.
2. A variety of tests specific to the client and based on individual characteristics, needs and requirements is preferable to any one single measure.
3. Minimum measurements should include weight, height, (calculated) BMI, and waist and hip circumference (calculated WHR).
4. Measurements should be carried out using standard protocols from recognised bodies such as the Society for Anthropometric Measurements or from the anthropometric standardised reference manual.
5. The validity, reliability and interpretation of all tests carried out should be known and, if required, related to the person being measured. This is especially important for the more high tech measurements such as BIA and NIR.
6. All measurement should, where possible, relate to appropriate norms within the population and ethnic group being tested. Where these are not available, 'next best' norms should be used with the possible inadequacies of this being explained to the client.
7. Care should be taken to ensure equivalent levels of hydration and digestion at different measurement periods (especially for BIA measures).
8. Body fat percentages should not be inferred from skinfold measures with very overfat or obese people.
9. Clients should be discouraged from weighing themselves too frequently (i.e. more than once per 1–2 week), because of the effect of fluid changes on body weight.

# IV
# CAUSES

# 7

# Influences on overfatness and obesity

SUMMARY OF MAIN POINTS

- The treatment of obesity has had only limited success and attempts at prevention have been a total failure.
- The traditional models for understanding obesity using simple energy balance may be partially responsible for these poor success rates.
- Scientific thinking in this area has evolved from simple physics, to biological and physiological ways of explaining the obesity.
- A new ecological paradigm is needed to incorporate the influences of biology, the environment and individual behaviour.
- The inclusion of physiological adjustment to changing energy stores in the model is also a key factor in understanding the dynamics of changing body fatness.
- The mediators through which the influences and moderators work are fat intake and fat utilisation in the body.

In spite of the huge personal expenditure on weight control, the burgeoning weight control industry, and the vast media attention given to the problem, it is obvious that all countries in the Western world are losing the battle of the bulge. One possible reason for this is that the issue may have been inadequately conceptualised in scientific terms. The failure to even stabilise the growth rate of obesity at the population level has led some health experts to suggest a paradigm shift in thinking about weight control. It has been claimed that all science progresses through 'paradigm shifts' in thinking where a paradigm is defined as '. . . the collective set of attitudes, values, procedures, techniques etc., that form the generally accepted perspective of a particular discipline at a particular time'.[1] In light of this, it is interesting to consider the evolution of thinking that has occurred in this area and to come up with a possible alternative, more all-encompassing approach on which better program planning—both prevention and treatment—can be based. This chapter considers three phases in the scientific thinking about weight control over recent years and proposes a new ecological model.

## SCIENTIFIC THINKING ABOUT WEIGHT CONTROL

### Traditional thinking: The physics model

It has always been thought that the main causes of excess body fat are simply too little exercise and/or too much food. The traditional model for defining this has been encompassed by the formula:

Change in energy stores = Energy Intake (EI) − Energy Expenditure (EE)
*where*

EI = calories from food

EE = resting metabolic rate (MR) + thermogenesis + daily physical activity

There are now a number of reports that have established this is clearly inadequate for describing weight gains and losses in living organisms.[2] According to the above calculation, for example, it has been estimated that a 75kg man who is in energy balance and who then adds an extra slice of toast and butter (100kcal) a day to his diet for 40 years would gain around 189kg over that time[3]—a prediction which is clearly not sensible. The discrepancy results because energy is more closely balanced in free living organisms than was once thought. This comes about because there are changes in EE and EI with changing weight (e.g. changes in metabolic rate and the energy cost of activity, or changes in food intake with changes in physical activity). The above formula then needs to be modified to reflect *rates* of change, thereby allowing for the effects of changing energy stores on energy expenditure (for more detail on adaptation see Chapter 14). It is now clear that initial differences between EI and EE (such as a modest increase in total calorie intake) do not lead to unbounded changes in body mass, hence the insufficiency of the physics approach.

## Adjustment in living systems: The biological model

To cater for the dynamic nature of energetics in living systems, a second phase of thinking in the field incorporated rates of change, i.e:

$$\text{Rate of change of energy stores} = \text{Rate of energy intake (EI)} - \text{Rate of energy expenditure (EE)}$$

The use of 'rates' in this equation allows for changes with time and hence allows for the effects of changing body mass on EE and EI. This would mean that a small change in energy balance (e.g. an increase in food) would not lead to a large increase in body fat because as body mass increases, there will be an increase in EE (through increased metabolic rate and the increased energy costs of moving a bigger body around). This will then balance the increased energy intake and the individual would thus again be in energy balance, although at a slightly higher body weight. Using this approach, it has been calculated that the extra slice of toast for the man mentioned above would only add around 2.7kg of weight over 40 years, which is clearly a much more realistic figure. This approach highlights the need to look for the cause of a chronic imbalance between energy intake and expenditure, rather than small, absolute differences of either one (which is the 'calorie counting' approach). However, this model still offers no clues about what causes a chronic energy imbalance in the first place. For that, a further explanation became available in the 1980s.

## Fat balance: The physiological model

The next development examined the separate nutrient balance equations, i.e. fat, alcohol, carbohydrate and protein equations. In human physiology it became clear that fat imbalance was the main cause of energy imbalance. Hence the formula to describe this became the following:

Rate of change of *fat* stores = rate of *fat* intake − rate of *fat* oxidation. [4]

This developed from important physiological studies in the 1980s which found that in humans, fat stores come largely from dietary fat, and that under most conditions, fat balance equals energy balance.[5] As we saw in Chapter 5, it is only under unusual conditions that humans convert significant amounts of non-fat calories into fat for storage. This model then suggests fat imbalance as the primary cause of an imbalance between energy intake and utilisation. Hence, the approach is a major step forward because it moves away from regarding obesity as a pathological state in a 'normal' environment. Because the problem of obesity is so widespread in modern societies, it suggests that the opposite is almost certainly true, i.e. that the spectrum of body sizes from lean to obese represents the normal variations of physiology and, within a 'pathological' environment (which favours obesity), many more are at the obese end of the spectrum. However, there are still problems with this approach. The fat balance equation above describes the changes in fat stores that occur *within* a given individual over time. It is less clear how differences in body fat *between* individuals arise. Why is it that some people remain relatively lean when they seem to have the same sort of lifestyle as others who are overfat? It also fails to explain the differences in obesity prevalence between populations. To explain this requires an expanded approach.

### An alternative paradigm: The ecological model

Any complete understanding of obesity must take account of the differences both within and between individuals and populations, as well as the moderating physiological adjustments which occur as a result of changes in energy balance. This would mean a more ecological approach to the problem which implies a delicate balance between a wide variety of competing forces. The model shown in Figure 7.1 suggests that there are three main influences on equilibrium levels of body fat—environmental, biological and behavioural—and these are mediated through fat/energy intake (F/EI) and/or fat/energy expenditure (F/EE), but moderated by physiological adjustments to changes in energy balance.

The model shown in Figure 7.1 adds the biological, environmental and behavioural influences to an equation whose end point is 'equilibrium stores' of body fat. This is a dynamic relationship where fat stores 'settle', at least temporarily, until there is some change in components of the equation, after which physiological adjustment occurs, or a new equilibrium, or 'settling point', is

**Figure 7.1:  An ecological paradigm for understanding overfatness and obesity**

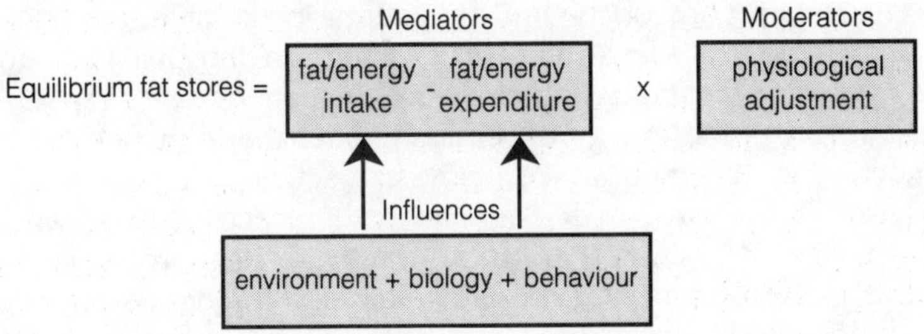

reached. This paradigm discards the notion of a 'set point' for body fat, whereby the body works to achieve and maintain a body fat mass of say 75kg. It also modifies the previous notions of energy balance by specifying the initial aspects of food, exercise, the rate of fat intake and the rate of fat utilisation respectively. Finally, the model incorporates the physiological adjustments which occur with body composition changes and which then bring it back into equilibrium. The components of the model are broken into the *mediators* (i.e. fat intake and expenditure), *influences* (environment, biology and behaviour) and the *moderators* (physiological adjustment); each of these are considered separately below but are then outlined in more detail as the basis of the remainder of this book.

## MEDIATORS

All of the effects of the influencing and moderating factors on body fat stores shown in Figure 7.1, are mediated through the final common pathway of food, or energy expenditure. In particular, the intake of energy through dietary fat, as we have seen in Chapter 5, and the utilisation of fat as energy through physical activity are now known to be the major influences on fat stores. However, as we have stressed the importance of fat in determining total energy, we now concentrate more on the two components of the energy balance equation as fat/energy intake (F/EI), and/or fat/energy expenditure (F/EE).

Nutritional components of fat and total energy intake are discussed in detail in Chapters 8–11. The most appropriate aspects of physical activity, which is the major modifiable component of EE for fat loss, are discussed in Chapters 12 and 13. The important point is the change in thinking about the components of energy balance from energy intake, to fat intake, and from energy expenditure to fat utilisation.

The implications of this on the energy intake side, are that it is much more realistic to aim for a change in the quality of the diet (reducing the fat:carbohydrate ratio) than by asking people to eat less. On the energy expenditure side, the approach places a much greater emphasis on 'physical activity', in contrast to 'exercise' for fat loss, and is in line with recent research which supports the use of lower duration, moderate intensity activity to achieve metabolic fitness[6] and promote fat loss. It redirects priorities for fat loss and obesity reduction away from a physical fitness orientation towards a strategy based on increasing low–moderate intensity activity (such as walking and 'incidental' exercise).

## MODERATORS

### Physiological adjustment

It has been recognised since the 1980s that overfeeding does not always result in the weight gain predicted by the physics energy balance equation. This is because in humans, the body defends itself against an imbalance between EI and EE by adjusting, within limits, the one to the other. Adjustment refers to the metabolic, physiological and behavioural changes that occur when the equilibrium, or 'settling point' is altered by a positive or negative energy imbalance. The adjustments tend to oppose the energy imbalance to minimise the effect on body weight changes. This helps to explain why, with such huge variations in energy intake and energy expenditure over a year, there are normally only minor fluctuations in body weight in most people. It also helps to explain the plateaus and rebounds during a fat loss program.

The popular belief (based on the physics model presented above) is that fat or weight loss can be calculated in a linear fashion from the calorie deficit. However, reducing the amount of food eaten over a set period by a total of 3500kcals, will not result in an automatic loss of 0.45kg of fat, which would be predicted as the storage equivalent of 3500kcal. Adjustment in energy expenditure through a decrease in metabolic rate in particular, would mean that the reduction in body stores is much less than expected. The opposite also holds true for a positive energy balance. When more is eaten than is used up as energy,

---

MYTH-INFORMATION
*Arguments about the benefits of butter or margarine are largely irrelevant when considering their use in fat loss. Both have equivalent fat energy value (i.e. 9 kcal/g).*

---

metabolic rate increases as body mass increases and again, the fat gain will be less than predicted.

It is this physiological adjustment which has been typically under-estimated in discussions of weight control, although a range of research has now identified it as a key factor in the long term failure of many programs.[7] Adjustment is a biological protective mechanism which prevents excessive long term gains and losses in body energy stores. It is more effective in some people than others (perhaps partly genetically determined). It may also be more strenuously invoked if the energy deficit and weight loss are large.

Adjustment occurs through a variety of mechanisms as summarised in Table 7.1. The short term adjustments are mainly through appetite control, although changes in the thermic effects of food (TEF) are directly related to meal size. Lethargy can be a marked feature of low energy intakes. In the longer term as fat mass and FFM decrease so do RMR and fat burning (higher RQ). Often the changes are greater than expected and this is called adaptation. For example, the fall in RMR may be much greater than expected for the loss of FFM. The adaptive changes are a sign of active mechanisms in the body opposing major shifts in body weight. Physiological adjustment and its implications for maintenance of fat losses after slimming, and in particular for dealing with plateaus in fat losses are discussed in more detail in Chapter 14.

## INFLUENCES

A major deficiency of previous paradigms of obesity has been their omission of factors which influence both extra- and intra-

**Table 7.1: Physiological adjustment to energy imbalances**

| Short term adjustments | Long term adjustments |
| --- | --- |
| • Appetite | • Resting metabolic rate (RMR) |
| • Thermic effect of food (TEF) | • Respiratory quotient (RQ) |
| • Level of exercise/spontaneous activity | |

**Figure 7.2: Environmental influences on obesity**

|  | Physical | Socio-cultural |
|---|---|---|
| Micro | | |
| Macro | | |

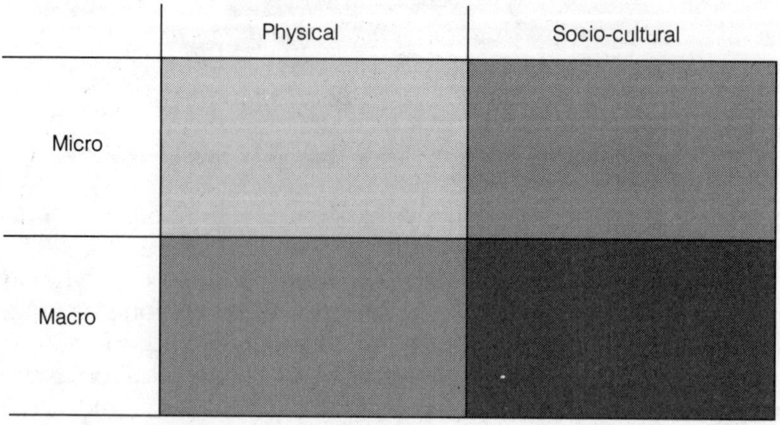

individual variations in energy balance—in particular the influence of environment, biology and behavioural factors on equilibrium body fat levels.

## Environmental influences

Abnormalities of biology or psychology cannot explain the big increases in obesity in modern societies. For this we need to look to the environment. Environmental influences on obesity occur either within a macro or micro environmental setting and can have either a physical or socio-cultural basis. This matrix of environments is illustrated in Figure 7.2.

Macro environmental influences at the physical level are those components of the larger world such as the food supply or technology. At the socio-cultural level, the macro environment represents population and community attitudes, values and norms. The micro environment refers to the immediate physical and social environments such as in the home, amongst peers and social contacts, pressures and attitudes in the family and immediate community. All of these environments can influence body fat levels through the mediation of energy intake or energy expenditure.

Environmental influences represent the public health arm of the obesity problem. While these exist, programs aimed at influencing behaviour at the individual level could only be expected to have limited effect. Any comprehensive approach to the prevention and treatment of overfatness and obesity must then consider both the macro and micro environments. Some ways of doing this are elaborated on in Chapter 15.

**Figure 7.3:   Biological influences on obesity**

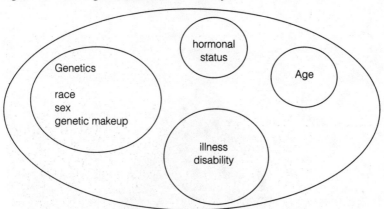

## Biological influences

Biological factors which influence body fat levels are generally not amenable to modification. The main biological factors known to influence obesity are genetic (including sex and race), age, hormone status, illness and disability (see Figure 7.3).

Heredity accounts for about 25–40 per cent of the variance of body mass index[8] suggesting that obesity has a strong genetic base, and according to evidence to date, is *polygenic* (influenced by many genes rather than a few). Sex differences are also known to affect fat/energy balance. In general, adipose stores are more hormonally controlled in females, particularly during the reproductive years.[9] Fat loss and maintenance of lower equilibrium fat stores also becomes more difficult with age. Differences occur between the sexes early in life, become greatest with the onset of menses, then tend to decrease with the changes in female hormone status in post-menopausal women. Finally, there is increasing evidence of racial influences on body composition.[10] The implications of these biological influences are in accepting factors beyond the wilful control of the obese person. Obesity should no longer be thought of as being due solely to either sloth and/or gluttony. Biological influences are discussed in more detail in Chapter 16.

## Behavioural influences

A third influencing variable, interacting with biological and environmental factors in the determination of body fat stores, is

**Figure 7.4:** **Behavioural influences on obesity**

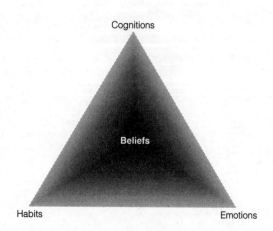

individual behaviour (Figure 7.4). Behaviour is the net result of complex psychological factors, involving the effects of habits, emotions and cognitions. Habits are learned ways of responding. Emotions represent the affective state of consciousness. Cognitive processes involve patterns of thinking. All of these are integrated by our belief systems about ourselves and the world. A common example of interactions between these factors is the vicious cycle of diet failure, guilt, depression, lowered self-worth and counter-productive habits which result from and lead to repeated failures with weight loss diet plans. Although there is no evidence to suggest that psychopathology is a major cause of obesity, these individual psychological factors have to be considered as having both a cause and effect association. Interventions designed to deal with these are a vital part of any overall strategy.[11]

These behavioural influences on overfatness and obesity are discussed in more detail in Chapter 17.

## ETHICAL ISSUES

The paradigm arising from previous models of obesity assumes that if an overfat person consults a professional or commercial weight loss organisation, he or she will be given a set of instructions which, if followed, will lead to an ideal body weight. Failure to achieve this is often attributed to sloth, gluttony or a lack of willpower. Under the new ecological approach presented here, it is acknowledged that an individual's equilibrium point is determined by a variety of influences, many of which are beyond his or her control. To lose body fat may be extremely difficult for people with the biological and environmental cards stacked against them. To achieve ideal body weight may be virtually impossible. So it becomes unethical to use extreme cases of weight loss and unrealistic goals of achievement as selling points for commercial weight loss programs. These are likely to give false expectations which may lead to cycles of failure, guilt and low self-esteem which can only be expected to magnify obesity and eating disorders. The ethical implications of this for fat loss programs are considered in more detail in Chapter 21.

## RE-DEFINING THE PROBLEM

As a working definition of obesity based on this new approach to the problem, we might consider the following:

> Obesity and overfatness result from the combined influences of the environment, behaviour and biology on increasing fat intake and reducing fat utilisation. Changes in body fat levels from their equilibrium or 'settling point' are moderated by physiological adjustments which temper the impact of fat/energy balance on body fat change.

## IMPLICATIONS

1. There is a need to recognise individual differences and, in particular, the influences of the environment, biology, behaviour and physiological adjustment in determining equilibrium body fat levels.
2. Distinguishing between different types of environments (micro, macro, physical, socio-cultural) is helpful for understanding the variety of external influences on an individual.
3. Obesity in modern society should be seen as a normal physiological response to a pathological environment rather than vice versa. For this reason, there is limited value in searching for abnormalities (genetic /metabolic/ psychological) as major causes of obesity.
4. There should be increased emphasis on influencing fat intake and fat oxidation as the modalities of first choice in managing and preventing obesity.

5. This approach heralds a move away from restrictive dieting and calorie counting, in favour of *ad libitum* lifestyle eating plans with an emphasis on a reduction in dietary fats.
6. It is necessary to emphasise the distinction between physical activity for fat loss (or prevention of fat gain) in contrast to 'exercise' for fitness.
7. Because of physiological adaptation, greater emphasis should be placed on long term maintenance of body *fat* losses in contrast to easier, short term, immediate changes in body *weight.*
8. It is ethically inappropriate to advertise or promote quick and large weight losses.
9. Because of the broad ranging requirements of the field of weight control management, its treatment belongs to no one particular profession. Hence, professionals must learn to work with and refer to experts in other disciplines in order to provide clients with the best opportunity to deal with their problems.

# V

# MEDIATORS—FAT/ ENERGY INPUT

# 8

# Dietary fat and how to reduce it

### SUMMARY OF MAIN POINTS

- Fat in food is a mixture of saturated, poly- and mono-unsaturated fatty acids, with different proportions in different foods.
- While saturated fats have the most detrimental effect on health, all fats and oils are currently thought to increase body fat.
- Reduction of fat should be the primary goal of any fat loss program, within a balanced diet.
- Client education should involve:
  - assessment of dietary fat intake for *obvious* as well as *hidden* fats
  - analysis of food choice and food preparation methods
  - recommended food selection and preparation for dietary fat reduction
  - information on how to read food labels and ingredient lists
  - explanation of nutritional claims about fat in foods.
- Reducing fats in the diet is the single most important factor for fat loss.

The nutritional issues covered in Chapters 8–11 are intended to highlight the nutritional mediating component considered in the model of obesity discussed in Chapter 7, (i.e. fat/energy intake).

As such, we will consider dietary fat and how to reduce it in detail in this chapter, then the alternative; increasing dietary carbohydrate and fibre in Chapter 9. Chapter 10 covers perspectives on hunger and appetite that are relevant to this recommended change in eating patterns and Chapter 11 is a critical review of some existing dietary programs. Reducing fat intake is regarded as an important part of a healthy eating pattern, but there is no attempt in this book to discuss all the aspects of healthy eating. There are several other specialist publications available for this.

## EATING FOR FAT LOSS

The trend highlighted in this book is away from 'dieting' and 'calorie counting' and in the direction of an 'eating plan' which is compatible with a long-term lifestyle change. In general, we will talk of *food selection* rather than a *diet*. In cases of obesity-related disease or extreme obesity, a restricted diet may be necessary, however the term 'diet' generally has negative connotations. Selecting appropriate foods with minimal restriction is a sensible goal for fat loss.

Eating for fat loss is essentially little different to that for eating for health, as described in the Healthy Eating Pyramid[1] shown in Figure 8.1. Food selection should focus on generous quantities of breads, cereals, fruits and vegetables; moderate amounts of protein such as meat, fish and dairy products; and only small amounts of fats, sugars and salt.

The emphasis in both fat loss and healthy eating plans is a reduction in dietary fat and an increase in complex carbohydrates and fibre. The Dietary Guidelines for Australians[2] shown in Table 8.1 are also applicable and should be incorporated into any total eating plan for fat loss. For more information on other aspects of eating for health, the reader is encouraged to consult other texts.[3]

The emphasis on a reduction in dietary fat does not disregard total energy. As we have described, fat intake is the main determinant of total energy intake.[4] However, minor reductions in

---

MYTH-INFORMATION

*Claims that cider vinegar breaks down fat are not true. The acid in vinegar does not even enter the bloodstream because it is neutralised by digestive juices.*

---

**Figure 8.1: The healthy eating pyramid**

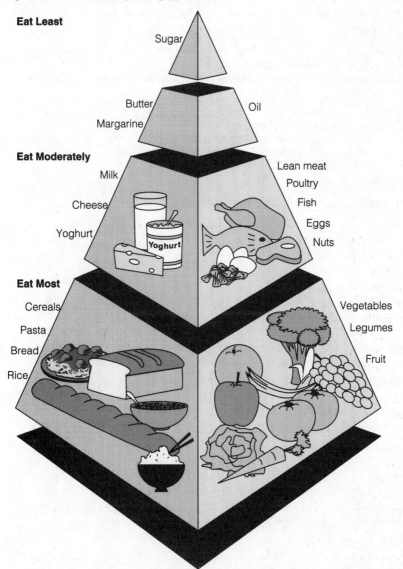

Source: The US Department of Agriculture (USDA) and the Department of Health and Human Services (DHHS) 1992

total fat and significant increases in other calories will lead to an overall increase in total energy and thus weight gain. This often happens when a person has been ingrained with the thinking that sugars, bread, potatoes and pasta are fattening. Those previously

113

'blacklisted' foods suddenly become good 'fat-free' foods and are over-eaten in large quantities.

**Table 8.1: Dietary guidelines for Australians**

1. Enjoy a wide variety of nutritious foods.
2. Eat plenty of bread and cereals (preferably wholegrain), vegetables, legumes and fruits.
3. Eat a diet low in fat, and in particular, low in saturated fat.
4. Maintain a healthy body weight by balancing physical activity and food intake.
5. If you drink alcohol, limit your intake.
6. Eat only a moderate amount of sugars, and foods containing added sugars.
7. Choose low-salt foods and use salt sparingly.
8. Encourage and support breast-feeding.

*Guidelines on specific nutrients*
1. Eat foods containing calcium. This is particularly important for girls and women.
2. Eat foods containing iron. This applies particularly to girls, women, vegetarians and athletes.

*Source:* NH&MRC

## RECOMMENDED FAT REDUCTIONS

Most recent research now shows the importance of dietary fat in causing increases in body fat.[5] National health targets recommend a reduction in the contribution of fat as a proportion of daily energy intake in adults to 30 per cent.[6] This is a conservative recommendation and takes into consideration what is realistic for individuals to achieve. Currently, fat contributes around 30–40 per cent of daily energy in most Western countries. To reduce fat to around 25 per cent of daily energy would require a fat intake of around 30–50g for most women and children; 40–60g for men; 70g for active teenagers and very active adults, and 80–100g for labourers or endurance athletes. Individuals with greater energy expenditures can obviously consume more fat and still be below the national target. Given what may be required for fat loss and available foods, a readily achievable and 'user-friendly' recommendation is to set the daily goal for fat intake at around 30–40g.[7] This is considerably less than the latest figures on mean dietary fat intake, which are at 93 and 74 grams per day for Australian men and women respectively.[8]

## MAIN FOOD SOURCES OF FAT

The major food sources of fat in the Australian diet as determined by the CSIRO Division of Human Nutrition are shown in Figure 8.2. The figures represent the average pattern of fat consumption

**Figure 8.2:** **Major food sources of fat in the Australian diet (as a proportion of total dietary fat intake)**

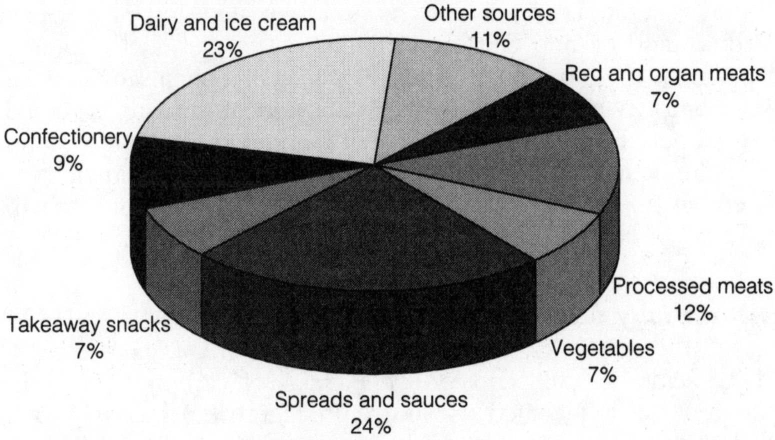

*Source:* CSIRO Division of Human Nutrition

by the Australian population. The personal pattern of fat intake will need to be considered when advising individuals about eating for fat loss.

## What is dietary fat?

Dietary fats or triglycerides are made up of three fatty acids joined together by a glycerol molecule. Oils are fats in liquid form and these have the same energy value (i.e. 9kcal/g) as 'hard' fats. Hence all fats and oils have been generally thought to have the same effect on body fat storage, although there is now some controversy about this.[9] In terms of other health issues such as blood cholesterol level, the *type* of fat is known to be more important.[10]

Fatty acids in foods can be divided into two major categories: saturated and unsaturated. Within the unsaturated category, there are also two major classes: monounsaturated and polyunsaturated.

**Table 8.2:** **Classification of dietary fats**

| Dominant fatty acid type | | |
|---|---|---|
| *Saturated* | *Unsaturated* | |
| | *Monounsaturated* | *Polyunsaturated* |
| Meat fats | Olive oil | Vegetable oils |
| Dairy fats | Canola oil | Some fish |
| Coconut oil | | |
| Palm kernel oil | | |

115

Fats in food contain a mixture of all types of fatty acids but in different proportions. For example, corn oil contains around 14 per cent saturated, 32 per cent monounsaturated and 52 per cent polyunsatured oil and butter contains about 52 per cent saturated, 23 per cent monounsaturated and 1 per cent polyunsaturated fat. It's a common misconception that only animal fats are saturated. Most plants and oils contain some saturated fat and in coconut and palm kernel oil, the saturated fats are the dominant ones (based on the fatty acid of greatest concentration). The dominant fatty acid in some common fats is shown in Table 8.2.

## What do fatty acids look like?

A fatty acid molecule consists of a chain of carbon atoms with hydrogen atoms attached as shown in Figure 8.3 below. (For a detailed description of fats and oils, other texts are available.[11]) The end of the molecule with three hydrogens (H) attached to the carbon (C) atom is called the *methyl* end. The other end is known as the *carboxyl* end. The chain has an even number of carbon atoms which stretches from four to 24 carbon atoms. If there are less than 8 carbons in the chain, the fatty acid is called a *short chain* fatty acid. *Medium chain* fatty acids have 8–10 carbons. If there are 12, 14, 16 or 18 carbons, it is called a *long chain* fat and these encompass most of the fatty acids in the human diet. These are commonly found in chocolate, meat and processed fats. Fatty acids with more than 20 carbons are *very* long chain fatty acids. They're found in breast milk, seafoods and some seeds and vegetables. Some medium chain fatty acids can be changed within the body to longer chain fatty acids.

**Figure 8.3:   Structure of a saturated fatty acid**

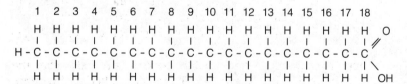

*Saturated fats*

If every carbon atom has its full complement of hydrogen atoms attached, the fat is *saturated*, meaning it has as many hydrogen atoms as it can possibly hold. The most commonly occurring saturated fatty acids have 10, 12, 14, 16 or 18 carbon atoms in

**Figure 8.4: Structure of a monounsaturated fatty acid—oleic acid (C18:n-9)**

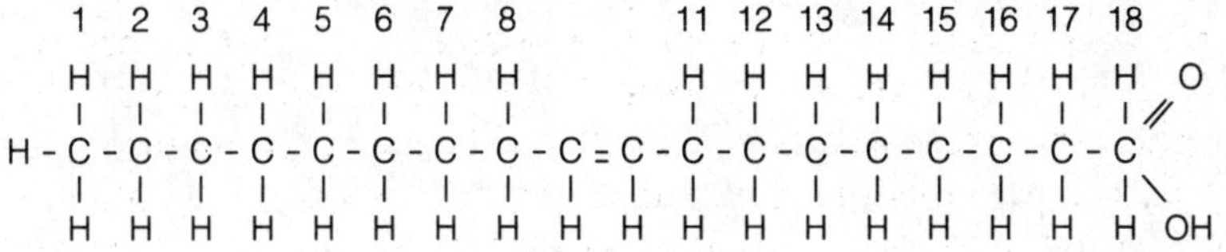

```
  1   2   3   4   5   6   7   8           11  12  13  14  15  16  17  18
  H   H   H   H   H   H   H   H           H   H   H   H   H   H   H   H   O
  |   |   |   |   |   |   |   |           |   |   |   |   |   |   |   |  //
H-C - C - C - C - C - C - C - C - C = C - C - C - C - C - C - C - C - C
  |   |   |   |   |   |   |   |   |   |   |   |   |   |   |   |   |   |  \
  H   H   H   H   H   H   H   H   H   H   H   H   H   H   H   H   H   H   OH
```

their chains and are found in meat fat, dairy fat, chocolate, processed fats, coconut and palm kernel oils. Increasingly, the saturated fat in our diet now comes in processed foods and originates from vegetable sources such as palm kernel oil.

Saturated fats are usually solid at room temperature (such as dripping, butter or chocolate). They keep fairly well and this makes them attractive to food manufacturers. They also make crisp biscuits and pastry and crunchy coatings on fried food. Because they're cheap, have a relatively long shelf life and are useful in processed foods, saturated fats are widely used by food manufacturers. Food labelling does not always indicate whether a fat is saturated or unsaturated.

### Unsaturated fats

There may be spots in the chain of carbon atoms making up a fatty acid where a carbon is not bound to the usual number of four hydrogen atoms. In such cases, the spare carbon forms a double bond with its neighbour. If there is only one double bond in the molecule, it looks like the molecule shown in Figure 8.4 and is called a *monounsaturated* fatty acid (MUFA). The most common monounsaturated fatty acid has 18 carbon atoms, with the double bond occurring on the 9th carbon atom from the methyl end of the chain. This is known as *oleic* acid. It is one of the most abundant fatty acids and is the principal fatty acid in olive and canola oils (called 'canola' for 'Canadian oil' to get around the embarrassing marketing problem of the term '*rapeseed*').

If there is more than one double bond in the fatty acid, the structure may look like Figure 8.5. These are called *polyunsaturated* fatty acids (PUFA). The most common source of PUFAs are oils such as sunflower, safflower, corn, sesame and soy bean.

### Omega-3 and Omega-6 fatty acids

Polyunsaturated fats are also categorised according to where the double bonds occur along the carbon chain. If the first double

**Figure 8.5: Structure of a polyunsaturated fatty acid—linoleic acid (C18:2n-6)**

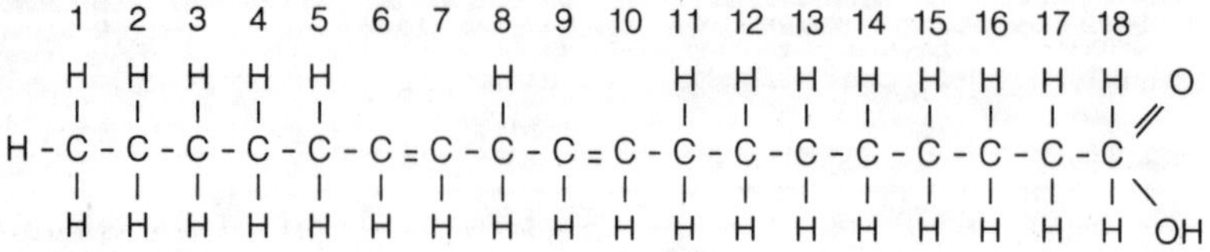

bond occurs on the third carbon from the methyl end of the carbon chain, the fatty acid is called an *Omega-3* fatty acid (also written as n–3). These polyunsaturated fatty acids occur in high concentrations in seafoods—especially oily fish, some seeds and breast milk. These have become popular lately as healthy oils which help prevent heart disease.[12] There is also now some evidence that they may not be converted to body fat as readily as other forms of dietary fat, although the research in this area is still in its early days. If the first double bond occurs on the sixth carbon from the methyl end of the chain, it is called an *Omega-6* fatty acid (also written as n–6). The polyunsaturated fatty acids in the vegetable oils mentioned earlier, and also in margarines made from these oils, are the Omega-6 type.

There are specific rules for describing fatty acids, according to their structure and the position of their double bonds. In the last example above, the double bonds occur on the sixth and ninth carbon atoms from the methyl end of the carbon chain. It would be written as C18: 2n-6 because it has 18 carbons (C18), two double bonds (:2) and the first double bond occurs on the sixth carbon from the end (n–6). The conventional notation is shown in Figure 8.6.

Omega-3s and Omega-6s are often in the news because nutritionists now believe they need to be present in the diet in the right balance. (Some of the products which come from the Omega-3 and Omega-6 fatty acids oppose each other in such complex processes as blood clotting and inflammation. This opposition keeps the balance between, for example, the blood clotting and blood thinning mechanisms.)

In many modern diets they are not well balanced, with many more Omega-6s than Omega-3s being eaten. The two major competitors are an Omega-6 fatty acid called *linoleic* acid (C18:2n–6) and an Omega-3 called *linolenic* acid (C18:3n–3): both are essential for humans. Linoleic acid definitely has advantages over the saturated fats for blood cholesterol, but too much of it will not only add to total fat intake, but may upset the balance between

**Figure 8.6:   Conventional naming of fatty acids**

Carbon length ⟶ **C18:2n-6 ⟶**  Location of first double bond from methyl end
Number of double bonds

Omega-6 and Omega-3. Rich sources of linoleic acid are vegetable oils and margarines. Rich sources of linolenic acid are fish and shellfish. Oleic acid (C18:n–9), the monounsaturated fatty acid found in olive and canola oils, has its only double bond on the 9th carbon from the methyl end of the chain. It does not compete with the other two essential fatty acids and is generally regarded as an all-round good guy in its effect on cholesterol and other metabolic processes, but it does add to total fat intake.

## Cis *and* trans *fatty acids*

To further complicate the picture, the unsaturated fats can be classified as *cis* or *trans* and this difference also has health effects. Fatty acids that contain a double bond can align themselves in two different geometric formations. If the hydrogen atoms attached to the carbons that have formed a double bond with each other are on the same side of the molecule, as shown in Figure 8.7, the molecule is called *cis*. If they are on opposite sides, they are called *trans*. The *cis* or *trans* configuration determines the fate of the molecule within the body.

The *trans* fatty acids are stiffer and tend to act more like saturated fat in the body, raising blood cholesterol levels. *Trans* fatty acids occur naturally (e.g. about 5 per cent in butter), or from processing (up to 15 per cent in margarine). The studies which have recently dulled the halo over polyunsaturated fats were done in the US and based on American diets in the 1970s when the harder 'stick' margarines were used. These are much higher in *trans* fatty acid content than the softer table margarines now in use.[13] Manufacturers are likely to lower the *trans* fatty acid content of foods even further in the future.

**Figure 8.7:   Structure of *cis* and *trans* fatty acids**

|  *Cis* fatty acid  |  *Trans* fatty acid  |
|---|---|
| H  H         H | H  H  H      H |
| I   I          I | I   I   I       I |
| C – C – C = C = C | C – C – C = C – C |
| I   I   I   I   I | I   I         I   I |
| H  H  H  H  H | H  H      H  H |

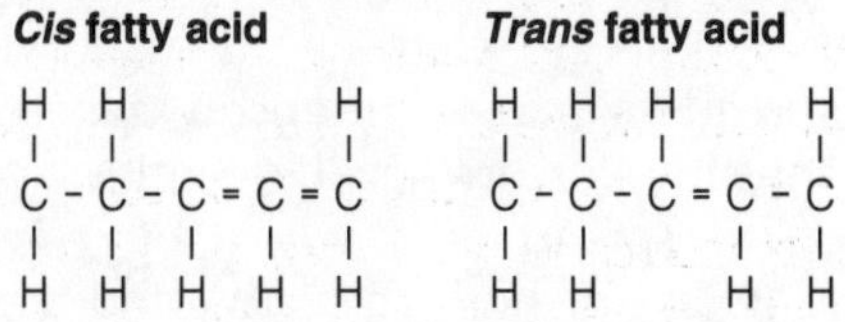

We have touched on a few of the metabolic consequences of the *type* of fat in the diet. As well as affecting blood cholesterol, clotting and inflammation, they may also affect other processes such as insulin and glucose metabolism and tumour formation. For body fat storage, the type of fat is of limited importance and the total amount of fat is still regarded as the most important.

## FATS, HEALTH AND FAT LOSS

It should be obvious from the discussion above that fats in food are not necessarily bad. In fact, a severe restriction of polyunsaturated fats may compromise the intake of essential fatty acids and vitamin E.[14] As the human body requires a minimum daily fat intake, it is neither wise nor practical to advocate a 'no-fat' diet.

The health implications of particular fats and oils are influenced by the proportion of different fats they contain. For example, olive oil is described as a *monounsaturated fat* but olive oil also contains polyunsaturated and some saturated fatty acids. Its *predominant* fatty acid is the monounsaturated *oleic* acid, so it is called monounsaturated. Margarines are often thought to be made up of polyunsaturated fats—in fact, about 20 per cent of the fat in these products is saturated fat. They also have some monounsaturated fatty acids and up to 15 per cent of the undesirable *trans* fatty acids. Their total polyunsaturated fat content makes up about half the fat they contain.

The percentage of different fatty acids is really only important if the total amount of fat in the food is significant. The fat content of both margarine and butter for example is about 80 per cent. This means that for every 100g they have 80g of total fat. One teaspoon—about the equivalent of a thin spread on a slice of bread—would contain about 4g of fat. About 30–40 per cent of the margarine will be cholesterol-raising fats (saturated plus *trans*) or about 1.5g per teaspoon. Butter, on the other hand, rates a high 60 per cent saturated and 5 per cent *trans* fatty acids in every 100g, or about 2.5g per teaspoon. The total fat content and the total energy in both products however are equal. By contrast, a food such as an egg has about 6g of fat, of which 2g is saturated (all of this in the yolk—egg white has no fat) which is midway between a thin spread of margarine and a thin spread of butter. The occasional consumption of small quantities of any of these foods (a teaspoon of spread or a whole egg) is likely to have little effect on the intake of both saturated and total fat. This fact

**Table 8.3: A summary of the characteristics of fats and oils**

Fats and oils have a number of variable components that alter their structure, function and effects on health. These include:

- The length of the carbon chain (*long*, *medium* or *short* chain fatty acids).
- The presence or absence of double bonds (*unsaturated* or *saturated* fatty acids).
- The number of double bonds (*mono-* or *poly*unsaturated fatty acids).
- The position of the double bond (*Omega-3*, *Omega-6* or *Omega-9* fatty acids).
- The position of hydrogen atoms on the same or opposite sides of the double bond (*cis* or *trans* fatty acids).

contrasts with common consumer beliefs regarding the perceived fat contents of margarine, butter and eggs.

One other postulated health implication is the susceptibility of fats to 'oxidise' (a chemical alteration to the fat molecule caused by reactions with oxygen 'free radicals'). Polyunsaturated fatty acids (PUFAs) are the most susceptible to oxidation, especially the long chain highly unsaturated Omega-3 fish oils (which is why fish 'goes off' faster than meat which contains mainly saturated fat). Balanced against this is the intake of anti-oxidants, especially vitamins C, E and beta carotene. Oxidised fats and other compounds in the body have been linked to many detrimental processes, including atherosclerosis, cancer formation, cataracts and ageing. Research is still intense in this area and many answers about oxidation and health effects are not yet available.

Monounsaturated fats (i.e. olive oil, canola oil, avocados) are generally seen as the best type of fat for health purposes. They tend to reduce blood cholesterol at least as well as the polyunsaturates, but don't oxidise as readily and have no known links with other health problems. In the case of olive oil, a major source of monounsaturated fat, we also have a long history of people safely consuming substantial amounts of it without apparent detrimental effects. Its major virtue may be not only that it contains a good mix of fatty acids, but that it also contains a wide variety of antioxidants. However, olive oil still contains the same energy, gram for gram, as other types of fats. And while there is some recent research now querying the fat storing potential of all fats, the prudent advice for those interested in lowering or maintaining body fat is still to decrease *all* fats in the diet.

## CLIENT EDUCATION: REDUCING FAT INTAKE

Given the above, the soundest and simplest component of a fat loss eating plan is to reduce dietary fat. To do this, we must consider the fat you can see (*obvious* fats) and the fats you can't

**Table 8.4: Short Fat Questionnaire (SFQ) for measuring fat intake**

*Short fat questionnaire*

1. How often do you eat fried food with a batter or breadcrumb coating?
   - Six or more times a week — 4
   - 3–5 times a week — 3
   - 1–2 times a week — 2
   - Less than once a week — 1
   - Never — 0

2. How often do you eat gravy, cream sauces or cheese sauces?
   - Six or more times a week — 4
   - 3–5 times a week — 3
   - 1–2 times a week — 2
   - Less than once a week — 1
   - Never — 0

3. How often do you add butter, margarine, oil or sour cream to vegetables, cooked rice or spaghetti?
   - Six or more times a week — 4
   - 3–5 times a week — 3
   - 1–2 times a week — 2
   - Less than once a week — 1
   - Never — 0

4. How often do you eat vegetables that are fried or roasted with fat or oil?
   - Six or more times a week — 4
   - 3–5 times a week — 3
   - 1–2 times a week — 2
   - Less than once a week — 1
   - Never — 0

5. How is your meat usually cooked?
   - Fried — 4
   - Stewed or goulash — 3
   - Grilled or roasted with added oil or fat — 2
   - Grilled or roasted without added oil or fat — 1
   - Eat meat occasionally or never — 0

6. How many times a week do you eat sausages, devon, salami, meat pies, hamburgers or bacon?
   - Six or more times a week — 4
   - 3–5 times a week — 3
   - 1–2 times a week — 2
   - Less than once a week — 1
   - Never — 0

7. How do you spread butter/margarine on your bread?
   - Thickly — 3
   - Medium — 2
   - Thinly — 1
   - Don't use butter or margarine — 0

8. How many times a week do you eat chips or French fries?
   - Six or more times a week — 4
   - 3–5 times a week — 3
   - 1–2 times a week — 2
   - Less than once a week — 1
   - Never — 0

9. How often do you eat pastries, cakes, sweet biscuits or croissants?
   - Six or more times a week — 4
   - 3–5 times a week — 3
   - 1–2 times a week — 2
   - Less than once a week — 1
   - Never — 0

l0. How many times a week do you eat chocolate, chocolate biscuits or sweet snack bars?

| | |
|---|---|
| Six or more times a week | 4 |
| 3–5 times a week | 3 |
| 1–2 times a week | 2 |
| Less than once a week | 1 |
| Never | 0 |

11. How many times a week do you eat potato crisps, corn chips or nuts?

| | |
|---|---|
| Six or more times a week | 4 |
| 3–5 times a week | 3 |
| 1–2 times a week | 2 |
| Less than once a week | 1 |
| Never | 0 |

12. How often do you eat cream?

| | |
|---|---|
| Six or more times a week | 4 |
| 3–5 times a week | 3 |
| 1–2 times a week | 2 |
| Less than once a week | 1 |
| Never | 0 |

13. How often do you eat more than a small serve of ice cream?

| | |
|---|---|
| Six or more times a week | 4 |
| 3–5 times a week | 3 |
| 1–2 times a week | 2 |
| Less than once a week | 1 |
| Never | 0 |

14. How many times a week do you eat more than a small piece of cheddar or other hard cheese, semi-soft cheese such as camembert or cream cheese?

| | |
|---|---|
| Six or more times a week | 4 |
| 3–5 times a week | 3 |
| 1–2 times a week | 2 |
| Less than once a week | 1 |
| Never | 0 |

15. What type of milk do you drink or use on breakfast cereal or in cooking?

| | |
|---|---|
| Condensed or evaporated | 4 |
| Full-cream | 3 |
| Full-cream and reduced-fat | 2 |
| Reduced-fat | 1 |
| Skim | 0 |

16. How much of the skin on your chicken do you eat?

| | |
|---|---|
| Most or all of the skin | 2 |
| Some of the skin | 1 |
| None of the skin/I am a vegetarian | 0 |

17. How much of the fat on your meat do you eat?

| | |
|---|---|
| Most or all of the fat | 2 |
| Some of the fat | 1 |
| None of the fat/I am a vegetarian | 0 |

**Scores:**

0–17: Your fat intake is relatively low. Focus on any problem areas.

18–39: Your fat intake is moderately high. Reducing fat in your diet will assist you with fat loss.

40+: Your fat intake is high. Reducing fat in your diet should be a high priority for fat loss.

---

*Reproduced with permission Professor Annette Dobson, Medical Statistics, University of Newcastle see (*hidden* fats). *Obvious* fats include butter, margarine, cooking oils, the fat on meat, and other visible fats. *Hidden* fats are those usually added to processed foods such as cakes, biscuits and potato crisps. Client education should involve an assessment of both these sources, plus information about lower-fat food options.

## Assessing dietary fat intake

A simple tool, the Short Fat Questionnaire (SFQ) developed by researchers at Newcastle University, can be used to assess dietary fat intake and provide education about sources of fat in the diet.[15] The SFQ gives an indication of habitual dietary fat intake from significant fat-containing foods. The SFQ provides an excellent check for *obvious* fats and some major food sources of *hidden* fats. When self-scored by totalling individual response scores, clients can become aware of their major sources of dietary fat and take steps to target those sources. As the SFQ measures 'habitual' intake of fat-containing foods rather than a 'single day' analysis, it targets eating practices that may have contributed to long term excessive fat consumption. The SFQ indicates a maximum score of 63, with a minimum score of zero. The SFQ is shown in Table 8.4 with score ratings for fat intake. The SFQ is obviously not meant to give a definitive measure of fat intake, but is useful in particular for measuring changes in people who have undertaken a low-fat eating plan. It is also necessary to be aware that for many people there is an 'eye-mouth' gap (not 'seeing' what they eat) and that reporting of actual food intake from a food intake questionnaire may need to be viewed cautiously.

A more specific analysis of fat intake can be performed using one of the many 'fat counters' available at most bookstores.[16] These provide a tool for identifying the fat content of a substantial number of foods. By performing a 'fat count' over a number of days, clients will become even more aware of their sources of dietary fat.

**Table 8.5: Information required on food labels**

1. The name of the product.
2. The name and address of the manufacturer, packer, importer or vendor.
3. The country of origin.
4. Ingredient list with ingredients listed in order of weight.
5. Identification of where the food was produced and a lot or batch number so the food can be traced to its packaging plant.
6. The date of packaging or a use by date.

**Table 8.6:   Nutrition information panels—a comparison**

| | Nutrition information per 100 g | |
| --- | --- | --- |
| | Food 1 | Food 2 |
| Energy | 2290 kJ | 1620 kJ |
| Protein | 6.1 g | 10 g |
| Fat | 37.1 g | 3 g |
| Carbohydrate | | |
| Total | 51.0 g | 81.1 g |
| Sugars | 0.4 g | 4.0 g |
| Dietary fibre | 5.6 g | |
| Sodium | 1600 mg | 670 mg |
| Potassium | 965 mg | 1230 mg |

## Reading food labels and nutrition information panels

The proliferation of readily accessible food items has led to a great deal of consumer confusion, especially when it comes to deciphering food labels and nutritional information panels.[17] There are food-labelling laws, although these are sometimes flouted by small manufacturers who attract less attention from food inspectors than larger manufacturers. Table 8.5 shows the information required on all food labels.

In addition to this, manufacturers are required to provide a nutrition information panel if any nutritional claim is made (e.g. low-fat, no added sugar). The panel must show protein, fat, carbohydrate (total and sugars), sodium, potassium and kilojoule content plus the quantity of any other nutrient for which a claim is being made.

In addition to providing lower-fat food options, clients should be educated about how to read food labels. This is particularly useful in interpreting the information on food packaging to reveal hidden fats in foods. The most important item to check on a nutrition information panel is fat content per 100g. Table 8.6 provides a per 100g comparison of panels for two foods, one with a high-fat and the other with a low-fat content.

Food 1 represents a packet of potato crisps, whereas Food 2 represents a packet of oven-baked pretzels. There is a big difference in fat content, and it is obvious the pretzel would be the better choice for a savoury snack. Although a figure for acceptable fat content is arbitrary and lower fat content is desirable, a figure of 10g of fat per 100g of food (or roughly 10 per cent fat by weight or less) provides a rough guide; that is, if a food contains more than 10g fat per 100g, its fat content is too high, and it should be avoided. It is also important to check that the

**Table 8.7: Commonly used names for fats in ingredient lists**

Lard, animal fat, animal shortening, coconut oil, palm oil, vegetable oil, butterfat, whole milk solids, copha, tallow, chocolate, chocolate chips, shortening, margarine, cocoa butter

**Table 8.8: Common ways of hiding fat in ingredient lists**

*Ingredients*: wheat flour, full cream milk powder, cocoa butter, sugar, cocoa liqueur, emulsifiers (322, 476), starch, colours (104, 110, 122, 133, 171), flavours

serving size is realistic. For example, a 200ml tub of regular yogurt will provide about 8g of fat, but if half a 1-litre container is consumed, this figure increases to 20 grams—half the recommended daily fat intake.

When a food product does not have a nutrition information panel, manufacturers are required to show ingredients by listing them in order of decreasing mass. When looking for fat in the ingredient list it is important to know that other substances may be equivalent to fat and to try to avoid foods that have fats near the beginning of the list (i.e. within the top three ingredients). Other common terms used for fats are shown in Table 8.7.

In order to disguise the amount of fat in some foods, manufacturers sometimes split the total fat content up into a number of fat components so that the main fat appears further down the ingredient list. The list in Table 8.8 shows how this can be achieved. The underlined ingredients mean 'fat'. Combining these and calling them 'fat' would require a move to the top of the list.

## Nutritional claims about fat

Nutritional claims on food packets can make food choices easier, saving time reading nutrition panels or doing complicated mathematical calculations, but the information must be correct, appropriate and reliable. Unfortunately, many claims are frequently misunderstood, misinterpreted or simply misread.[17] As a result of the consumer's perception of the nutritional content of foods, the Australian National Food Authority (NFA) has produced a Code of Practice on nutrient claims in food labels and in advertisements. Launched in 1995, after lengthy consultation with food manufacturers and health professionals, the Code provides clear criteria that manufacturers must meet before they are permitted to make nutritional claims. There is also a limitation on what claims can

**Table 8.9:   Nutritional claims about fat and what they mean**

| *What it says* | *What it means* |
|---|---|
| Reduced-fat<br>Lower fat<br>Less fat | The food must not contain more than 75 per cent of the total fat content of the same quantity of the regular item (reference food). |
| Low-fat<br>Low in fat | Not more than 3g total fat per 100g of food or 1.5g total fat per liquid food. If the claim is made for a food naturally or intrinsically low in fat, it must refer to the whole class of similar foods. For example, a 'low-fat' claim for pasta must note that 'pasta is a low-fat food'. |
| Fat-free | No more than 0.15g of fat per 100g of food. |
| % fat-free | The food must meet the requirements for 'low-fat' and must carry a statement of the actual fat content (expressed as a percentage of the food) close to the claim. |
| % free | Cannot be used to refer to any other nutrient other than fat. |
| Lite or light | The characteristic which makes the food light must be stated on the label. The term may not necessarily apply to fat content, but rather colour or flavour. |
| Diet | This claim most often applies to foods which have an energy content significantly lower than that at which a 'reduced-energy' claim can be made. Unless other criteria are met the food must:<br>• have an energy content not more than 60 per cent of the reference food<br>• have a reduced energy content of at least 40 kcal per 100g of food (20kcal per 100g of liquid food)<br>• there must be a statement of comparison with the reference food. |

*Source:*   National Food Authority

be made and on which foods.[18] Table 8.9 provides a summary of the NFA's permitted claims and the criteria for these.

## METHODS OF REDUCING DIETARY FAT INTAKE

The methods by which individuals select low-fat diets have been placed into four categories.[19] Table 8.10 provides an explanation of these methods with examples. A comprehensive approach to reducing dietary fat will consider ingredients, cooking methods, different foods and reduced-fat foods.

Another method often promoted for fat loss is the fill, trim, pick, nick and skip technique,[20] i.e.:

*Fill:*  Fill your diet with low-fat foods (fill your plate with vegetables, fill out your meatloaf with bread crumbs, fill up on bread and fruit).

*Trim:*  Trim the high-fat bits (trim fat from meat, remove chicken skin, scrape the butter off the cafeteria muffin and the cream off the sponge).

127

**Table 8.10: Methods for reducing dietary fat**

1. *Exclusion—eliminating certain foods or food preparation techniques:*
   - not putting butter or margarine on toast
   - avoiding sausages and luncheon meats
   - eating salads without mayonnaise or dressing
   - avoiding fried foods

2. *Modification—altering foods to be lower in fat:*
   - trimming fat off meat
   - grilling rather than frying
   - skimming fat off soups
   - draining fat off cooked mince

3. *Substitution—using reduced-fat or low-fat varieties of regular foods:*
   - choosing reduced-fat cheeses
   - having skim milk instead of full-cream milk
   - using lean mince
   - eating reduced-fat ice cream

4. *Replacement—changing to new foods or ingredients:*
   - swapping lemon juice for salad dressing
   - eating yoghurt for dessert instead of ice cream
   - having fruit for a snack rather than a piece of cake
   - basting meats with vegetable stock and not oil

*Pick:* Pick the low-fat foods (low-fat milk, yogurt instead of sour cream, fruit instead of cake, low-fat salad dressings).

*Nick:* Just nick those high-fat foods. Be a gourmet (who takes a little, treasuring the taste) not a gourmand (who takes a lot and treasures the volume).

*Skip:* Skip the high-fat foods more often. Have takeaways once in a while, not every week. Eat chocolate and desserts only on special occasions.

Any combination of fat-related dietary changes can lead to a target level of fat intake. Research has shown that substitution of low-fat foods such as reduced-fat dairy products is more easily adopted and maintained than the avoidance of high-fat items like meats and savoury snacks.[21] It appears that people are willing to avoid some 'fatty' foods and limit consumption of others. Distinguishing between food items a client is willing to exclude, and those they are willing to limit intake of will be important when assessing individual eating behaviour.

Some research has been carried out to examine the individual perceptions of fat content in foods. In one study, men and women were asked to estimate the fat content of various foods. The results showed that for some foods the fat content was dramatically under-estimated, whilst for other foods it was over-estimated. Foods commonly mis-classified as being higher in fat included potato, spaghetti, baked beans and beer. Those foods incorrectly perceived to be lower in fat included chicken with the skin, sardines, cheese and peanuts. Almost 70 per cent of subjects thought that margarine was lower in fat than butter.

Even doctors and nutritionists studied in this survey had widely varying perceptions of fat in foods. These findings underpin the inability of consumers to recognise the fat content of their own diets and the need to educate clients about the fat content of foods.[22]

From all of the above, it appears obvious that fat is *the* key nutrient for reducing body fat because (a) it is higher in energy density than other nutrients, (b) it is stored more efficiently as fat in the body and (c) it is less likely to result in 'fullness' after a meal and therefore to encourage a greater food intake. However, caution needs to be taken with some people who are restrained eaters and who see food labels in black and white terms. This was demonstrated in one study where non-dieting women were given yoghurt to eat 30 minutes before a meal, and were told it was either high-fat or low-fat. When they were told it was low-fat they tended to eat more at the following meal, hence perhaps negating the effect of the reduced-fat product.[23] Hence, although prime attention needs to be given to fat in the diet, attention should not be distracted from total energy input and compensations which may occur.

## IMPLICATIONS

1. A reduction in dietary fat will be the prime objective of any fat loss eating plan.
2. Calorie counting should be avoided in favour of a low-fat eating plan.
3. Fat reduction should be recommended only in the context of a balanced diet.
4. Although some fats may have better health value than others, it is currently prudent to recommend a decrease in all dietary fats for body fat reduction.
5. A 'user-friendly' rule is to try to reduce total daily fat intake to below 40g. Even so, any reduction will be moving in the right direction.
6. Clients can identify sources of dietary fat using the Short Fat Questionnaire.
7. A 'fat count' may be a useful exercise to identify more specific sources of dietary fat.

8. Clients should be taught to read food labels, nutrition information panels and ingredient lists to assist the appropriate selection of foods.

9. Clients should be encouraged to eat regular servings of low-fat foods.

10. Spreads such as butter and margarine may be easily minimised or eliminated.

11. The use of oils should be minimised.

12. Clients should be taught low-fat cooking and food preparation procedures.

13. Help clients to determine which food sources of fat they are willing to exclude and which ones they are willing to limit in quantity.

14. Any low-fat eating plan prescribed for fat loss must be one that can be comfortably adhered to for a lifetime.

15. Although of secondary importance to dietary fat reduction, total energy input may need to be reduced if desired fat loss is not achieved with dietary fat reduction alone.

# 9

# Dietary carbohydrate and how to increase it

SUMMARY OF MAIN POINTS

- A low-fat diet has an automatically high percentage of carbohydrate.
- Carbohydrate is most simply classified as either sugar, starch or fibre.
- More complex classifications are currently being developed.
- A high-carbohydrate intake has not been linked to obesity in populations.
- A reduction in sugar consumption may be wise for some individuals.
- Client education should involve:
  — assessment of dietary carbohydrate intake and its specific components; sugar, starch and fibre
  — recommended food selection for increasing dietary fibre
  — information on how to read food labels and ingredient lists
  — explanation of nutritional claims about carbohydrate in food

Until recently, carbohydrates have drawn far less scientific attention than dietary fat. Now there is ample evidence to show that specific components of carbohydrate are beneficial for both health and body fat management. In percentage terms, carbohydrate will replace fat in the diet if a lower-fat eating plan is adopted. This chapter describes carbohydrate, the new dimensions of its role and the implications for client education.

## WHAT IS CARBOHYDRATE?

Carbohydrate is the term given to a group of macronutrients which contain carbon, hydrogen and oxygen combined in a unique way. Carbohydrates can be small or large molecules, depending on the number of structural units from which they are made. Carbohydrate is therefore not a single entity, but a group of substances with major chemical and nutritional differences.[1] The classification of carbohydrates is not uniformly agreed upon, but the strict chemical classification breaks them into monosaccharides, disaccharides, oligosaccharides and polysaccharides, depending on the number of sugar units. However, for simplicity and practicality, it is still probably best to consider three major categories of interest: sugars, starches and fibre.[2]

### Sugar

Sugars, which are often called 'simple sugars', are made up of only one or two structural units. Monosaccharides (*mono* meaning one and *saccharide* meaning sugar) are made up of a single carbon ring. These include glucose, fructose and galactose. Glucose is the major monosaccharide in the body and is also known as dextrose or blood sugar; fructose is found in fruits and galactose is only present by itself in nature in very small amounts. Two monosaccharides joined together are called a disaccharide (*di* meaning two). These include maltose, sucrose and lactose. Maltose is present in sprouting grains and is made up of two glucose units bonded together. Sucrose, more commonly known as table sugar, consists of glucose and fructose. Lactose consists of glucose and galactose and is the sugar present in mammalian milk. A schematic representation of the structure of glucose and sucrose is shown in Figure 9.1.

### Starch

A carbohydrate containing many monosaccharide units is called a polysaccharide (*poly* meaning many) or starch. More commonly known as 'complex carbohydrates' these are the storage forms of carbohydrate in plants—amylose and amylopectin. Figure 9.2 shows a portion of the complex, branched structure of starch.

**Figure 9.1:   Structure of sugars**

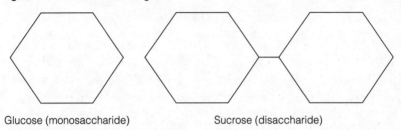

Glucose (monosaccharide)                              Sucrose (disaccharide)

**Figure 9.2:   Structure of starch**

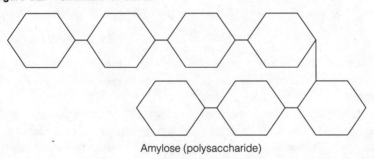

Amylose (polysaccharide)

## Fibre

Contrary to popular belief, fibre is not just one substance. Rather, the term is an all-embracing one for a number of components found in plants, which include cellulose and other *insoluble* fibre components and gel-forming or *soluble* fibres such as pectins, gums and mucilages found in fruits, oats and barley.[3] All fibre is made up of multiple saccharide units and nutritional scientists now prefer to call fibre a non-starch polysaccharide (NSP). Table 9.1 summarises the classification of fibre with examples of food sources.

## WHAT HAPPENS TO CARBOHYDRATE IN THE BODY?

Before examining the health and fat loss benefits of carbohydrates it is essential to take a brief look at how carbohydrates are digested and absorbed in the human body. First we need to start with the gastrointestinal tract (GIT). The GIT is a long tube stretching from the mouth to the anus. The digestion of carbohydrate starts in the

**Table 9.1:  Classification of fibre**

| Category | Insoluble | Soluble |
|---|---|---|
| Substances | cellulose<br>hemicelluloses | pectins<br>gums<br>mucilages |
| Examples of<br>food sources | wheat bran<br>processed bran<br>vegetables | oat bran<br>barley<br>fruits |

mouth, where enzymes in saliva start to break some of the bonds between saccharide units. After swallowing, carbohydrate enters the stomach ready to be released into the small intestine in small quantities. In the small intestine various enzymes perform the major part of carbohydrate digestion by breaking the bonds and releasing monosaccharides for absorption. Once absorbed, carbohydrate, in the form of glucose or fructose, goes to the liver where it is stored or put into the bloodstream as blood glucose for energy production or for storage in the muscles as glycogen.

Dietary fibre meets a somewhat different fate. Most fibre resists the digestive enzymes of the intestine and passes through to the large bowel. Here, some of it is metabolised by bacteria that produce the specific enzymes necessary for breakdown. This process is known as 'colonic fermentation'. The end products include the gases carbon dioxide, methane and hydrogen along with volatile fatty acids called short chain fatty acids (SCFAs). The SCFAs are absorbed from the large bowel, enter the bloodstream and are transported to the liver. The degree of fermentation in the large bowel depends on the type of fibre and varies between individuals. This explains why some people produce a lot of gas and others produce very little following consumption of fibre-rich foods.[4] Soluble fibres are entirely digested by bacteria and produce most of the SCFAs. Insoluble fibres are digested to only a small degree and the amount depends on the time spent in the large bowel before excretion.

The term *resistant starch* is a relatively new addition to the fibre scene. This is used to describe polysaccharides which are resistant to normal enzymatic digestion. This means that a portion of the starch eaten in foods will pass through the stomach and small intestine to the large bowel where it is fermented in a similar way to fibre. For this reason most nutritionists currently regard resistant starch as a component of dietary fibre. Resistant starch can occur naturally, such as in raw potato or bananas, be formed in partly milled grains and seeds, or can form following heating

**Table 9.2: Approximate resistant starch content of specific foods**

| Food | Resistant starch (g/100g of dry food) |
|---|---|
| White and wholemeal bread | 1 |
| Corn flakes | 3 |
| Porridge oats | 2 |
| Rye crispbread | 3 |
| Potato boiled, hot | 5 |
| Potato boiled, cool | 10 |
| Spaghetti, freshly cooked | 5 |
| Peas, cooked | 5 |
| Haricot beans, cooked | 18 |

*Source:* Englyst and Kingman 1992[5]

and cooling of cooked potatoes, bread and cornflakes.[5] Table 9.2 shows the approximate resistant starch content of specific foods. Food manufacturers have been able to incorporate resistant starch into white bread and other foods without affecting the sensory qualities of texture and flavour. This is a major advantage as consumers can eat foods that are higher in this fibre-like substance, but not radically different from more accepted forms.

This new dimension in carbohydrate physiology has stimulated another broad classification of carbohydrates. Nutritional scientists now use the terms 'available' (sugars and most starches) and 'unavailable' (resistant starch and fibre) when referring to the nutritional implications of carbohydrates.

## THE GLYCAEMIC INDEX

Starches, because of their more compound nature, have been thought to be more slowly digested and therefore to offer great benefits in the treatment of disease such as diabetes and for fat loss. However, recently it has been shown that digestion and metabolism are not that simple. The speed with which carbohydrates are broken down and absorbed is not simply determined by whether they are 'simple' or 'complex' and another measure has been developed to classify this.

The Glycaemic Index (GI) is a method of classifying the

---

### MYTH-INFORMATION

*Contrary to popular belief, potatoes, bread and other starchy foods have a low potential for increasing body fat. These contain virtually no dietary fat and their high carbohydrate level is useful for energy.*

---

glycaemic (i.e. blood sugar) response to carbohydrate-rich foods. Put another way, it is a measure of how quickly carbohydrate reaches the bloodstream. Foods can be tested and ranked according to a measure of their GI. Figure 9.3 shows a comparison of blood glucose levels for glucose and lentils during a GI test. The GI is calculated by measuring the area under the curve (of glycaemia) versus time, after consuming a food containing 50g of available carbohydrate by comparison with 50g of reference food (either glucose or white bread). Blood glucose testing is carried out every 15–30 minutes for 2–3 hours. The GI is then calculated using the formula:

$$GI = \frac{\text{blood glucose area of the test food}}{\text{blood glucose area of a standard food}} \times 100$$

The lower the GI of a food, the flatter the curve of blood glucose response, meaning the slower this is digested and converted to blood sugar.

It does not necessarily follow that all sweet sugary foods will be quickly absorbed and therefore have a high GI. It is much more complex and depends on a number of characteristics of the food consumed,[6] e.g.:

*Type of sugar*—Glucose (GI = 100) has a higher GI than fructose (GI = 20). Temperate fruits (e.g. apples, pears, oranges) have a higher fructose content and therefore lower GI than tropical fruits (e.g. watermelon, rockmelon, mangoes).

*Nature of the starch*—The ratio of two types of starches (amylose:amylopectin) can affect the GI of foods. Amylopectin is more easily digested than amylose. Therefore, foods such as legumes, with a high amylose:amylopectin ratio have a lower GI than rice which has a higher amylopectin content.

*Processing and particle size*—Food particle size is a determinant of GI. This is shown with bread processing. Wholemeal bread has a finer texture than rye bread and thus a higher GI.

*Cooking methods*—Cooking affects the degree of gelatinisation of fruits and thus GI. Stewed fruits have a higher GI than fresh fruits.

*Starch–nutrient interactions*—Carbohydrate forms molecular complexes with fats and proteins. This happens, for example, in a baked cake where GI will be reduced.

*Fat*—Large amounts can reduce GI (e.g. in ice cream) and hence high-fat foods may have a desirable GI but still be undesirable in terms of energy content.

**Figure 9.3: Glycaemic Index response**

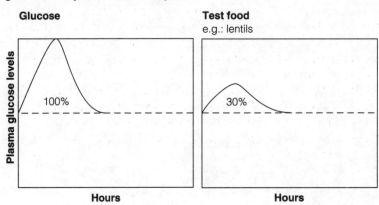

Glucose

Test food
e.g.: lentils

*Fibre*—This depends on type of fibre. Insoluble fibre appears to have no immediate effects. However, soluble fibre (e.g. guar gum) can decrease the rate of absorption of glucose and hence decrease GI. Fibre supplements will not have the same effect because the fibre is not packaged into the food. Resistant starch will also lower the GI of a food.

Taking these properties into account we can see why, in Table 9.3, wholemeal bread has a higher GI than rye bread and a pineapple has a higher GI than an apple. GI is not a simple function of the sugar content of foods and detailed tables showing the GIs of a wide variety of foods are now available.[7]

There are day-to-day variations in GI due to physiological effects, and the GI of component foods can predict the likely effect of a meal.[8] Sydney University studies have shown that low-GI foods may be beneficial for fat loss as they decrease hunger ratings. Due to the slower absorption of low-GI foods, they may result in less rapid fluctuations in blood glucose and appetite changes for some individuals.[9]

Australian researchers are leading the world in GI research. For more information on this evolving topic, please refer to *The GI Factor* by Sydney University's Professor Jennie Brand Miller.[10]

## CARBOHYDRATES, HEALTH AND FAT LOSS

There is considerable scientific backing for the health benefits of a diet with a high proportion of starches. National health targets suggest that carbohydrates should provide about 55–60 per cent of daily energy. Unfortunately, carbohydrate intake in most Western

**Table 9.3:  Glycaemic Index of selected foods**

| Low GI (below 55) | Intermediate GI (55–70) | High GI (more than 70) |
|---|---|---|
| Carrot (49) | Arrowroot biscuits (69) | Cornflakes (77) |
| Grapefruit (25) | Pineapple (66) | Rice Bubbles (89) |
| Apple (36) | Raisins (64) | Watermelon (72) |
| Rye bread (50) | Honey (58) | Bagel (72) |
| Spaghetti (41) | Sweetcorn (55) | Brown rice (76) |
| Sponge cake (46) | Basmati rice (58) | Calrose rice (83) |
| Baked beans (48) | Taco shells (68) | Broad beans (79) |
| Lentils (29) | Sucrose table sugar (65) | Baked potato (85) |
| Yoghurt (33) | Wheatmeal biscuits (62) | Glucose (100) |
| Fructose (23) | Sao biscuits (70) | Parsnip (97) |
| Peanuts (14) | Shortbread biscuits (64) | Corn chips (72) |
| Potato crisps (54) | Orange juice (57) | Wholemeal bread (77) |
| All Bran (30) | White bread (70) | Jelly beans (80) |

*Source:*  Brand Miller, Foster-Powell and Colaguri, 1996[10]

countries has declined this century with the increased consumption of fat.[2] Fibre intake in most Western countries averages only about half the national target of an achievable 30g per day.

The first idea that fibre could protect against certain diseases appeared in 1960, when researchers observed that the degenerative illnesses common in affluent societies were rare in rural Africa where diets were high in unrefined plant foods.[11] Subsequent studies confirmed the health properties of fibre and it is now considered to have a role in protection against chronic diseases such as cardiovascular disease, colo-rectal cancer, and the management of constipation and diabetes. The specific benefits depend on the type of fibre. Foods high in *insoluble* fibre reduce transit time (i.e. shorten the time for food to pass through the GIT), soften stools by holding water and increase stool volume. In contrast, foods high in *soluble* fibre have little effect on bowel transit but appear to slow the rate of carbohydrate absorption due to their gel-forming ability. This helps to reduce rapid fluctuations in blood glucose and insulin among people with diabetes.

The combination of the effects of different fibres (including resistant starch), the SCFAs produced and a diet low in fat are all thought to protect health, so it has been difficult to credit any one factor. Nutritionists therefore recommend a diet low in fat with a variety of foods containing all types of starch and fibre.

A low intake of carbohydrate in any form appears to be linked to obesity on a population level[12] because, by default, it is a high-fat diet. The claim that carbohydrates, whether as sugars or starches, are 'fattening' is a myth. However, it is prudent for some individuals who are obese and who consume large quantities of sugars, to moderate their intake as a second level of priority after decreasing fat.

## CLIENT EDUCATION: INCREASING FIBRE INTAKE

The specific component of carbohydrate we are seeking to increase is fibre. By selecting meals and snacks with a greater fibre content, individuals are likely to increase the intake of starches. As will be explained in Chapter 10, increasing fibre intake also minimises the risk of hunger when eating less fatty foods.

A gradual increase in fibre intake should be recommended. This will minimise possible side effects which include flatulence and possibly diarrhoea. When increasing fibre intake, also check fluid intake. If fluid intake is inadequate, constipation may result due to absorption of water by fibre in the large bowel.

It is also wise to caution clients against an excessive fibre intake. Besides the obvious gaseous effects, large quantities of

**Table 9.4: Rating fibre intake**

Add all the points scored daily using the point rating chart below.

| Food | Serving size | Points |
|------|-------------|--------|
| Wholegrain cereal | 1 metric cup (1 medium bowl) | 4 |
| Other cereal | 1 metric cup (1 medium bowl) | 1 |
| Wholegrain bread | 1 slice (1/2 roll) | 2 |
| White bread | 1 slice (1/2 roll) | 1 |
| Fruit | 1 medium piece (1 cup berries/cherries) | 3 |
| Potato (with skin) | 1 medium | 2 |
| Rice, brown | 1 cup cooked | 3 |
| Rice, white | 1 cup cooked | 1½ |
| Pasta, wholegrain | 1 cup cooked | 8½ |
| Pasta, white | 1 cup cooked | 3½ |
| Baked beans | 1 cup canned | 8 |
| Unprocessed bran | 1 tablespoon | 2 |
| Small side salad | | 4 |
| Cooked vegetables | per vegetable | 2 |

*Daily fibre rating. Enter your score daily*

| Mon | Tues | Wed | Thurs | Fri | Sat | Sun |
|-----|------|-----|-------|-----|-----|-----|
| | | | | | | |

Total score for the week =

*Rating*
5 or more days more than 30 points . . . *Excellent*
5 days around 20–30 points . . . *Average*
5 days less than 20 points . . . *Lots of room for improvement*

insoluble fibre—particularly wheat bran—can interfere with the absorption of iron by the body.

## Assessing dietary fibre intake

A 'fibre count' can be performed to identify sources of fibre and opportunities for increased intake. A greater fibre intake will result from increased consumption of fruits, vegetables, wholegrain cereals, legumes and other unprocessed plant foods. Client education should promote an eating style which includes these foods. A typical fibre check test, with grams of fibre represented as 'points', is shown in Table 9.4. As this list is limited to major fibre-containing foods, it can only provide a rough estimate of dietary fibre eting habits. More detailed lists can be found in most 'fat counter' books.

## Reading food labels for carbohydrates

Nutrition information panels indicate carbohydrate content by showing the 'total carbohydrate' and the quantity of 'sugars' per 100g. The starch content can be calculated by subtracting sugars from the total. Table 9.5 provides a comparison between white and wholemeal bread. Both breads contain a relatively large amount of starch—44.4g and 40.7g respectively. Although technically carbohydrate, fibre content is shown separately. As you would expect, wholemeal bread contains more fibre.

In the absence of a nutrition information panel, an ingredient list can give an indication of the fibre content of a food. Names such as wholewheat, bran, wheatbran, wholegrain, wheatgerm, wheatmeal and oatbran appearing near the front of an ingredient list may indicate a generous fibre content.

An ingredient list can also provide an indication of sugar

**Table 9.5:** Nutrition information panels for two types of bread

|  | White | Wholemeal |
|---|---|---|
|  | Per 100g | Per 100g |
| Energy | 1037kJ | 1000kJ |
| Protein | 8.9g | 9.4g |
| Fat | 2.4g | 2.5g |
| Carbohydrate |  |  |
|    Total | 46.8g | 43.0g |
|    Sugars | 2.4g | 2.3g |
| Dietary fibre | 3.0g | 6.8g |

**Table 9.6: Nutritional claims about fibre and what they mean**

| What it says | What it means |
|---|---|
| Source of fibre<br>Contains fibre | The food must contain at least 1.5g total fibre per serving of food. |
| High-fibre<br>High in fibre<br>Good source of fibre | At least 3g total fibre per serving of food. |
| Very high in fibre<br>Excellent source of fibre | At least 6g total fibre per serving of food. |
| Increased fibre<br>Fibre-enriched<br>More fibre | At least 3g total fibre per serving of food. This claim can only be used for foods which had at least 1.5g of fibre prior to enrichment. There must also be a statement of comparison with a reference food. |
| Added fibre | Must meet the 'high-fibre' claim, with a statement of comparison. |

*Source:* National Food Authority

content. Sugar can be identified by numerous other names: sucrose, maltose, lactose, dextrose, fructose, glucose, sorbitol, mannitol, glucose syrup, corn syrup, golden syrup, disaccharides, monosaccharides, polysaccharides, modified carbohydrate, raw sugar, brown sugar, molasses, honey and treacle.

## Nutritional claims about carbohydrates

Like fat, there are requirements for manufacturers' claims about fibre in food. Table 9.6 shows permitted claims and what they mean.

### METHODS FOR INCREASING DIETARY FIBRE INTAKE

An increase in dietary fibre will occur as fat-containing foods are

**Table 9.7: Methods for increasing dietary fibre**

- Use wholegrain bread and cereals such as brown rice, wholemeal spaghetti and other pasta, wholegrain breakfast cereal, wholegrain crispbread, oatmeal or wholemeal porridge, wheatmeal biscuits, wholemeal flour and other wholegrain cereal foods.
- Eat at least three pieces of fruit and four serves of vegetables each day.
- Eat the skins on fruits and vegetables e.g. potatoes in their jackets and the skins on apples, pears, peaches, etc.
- Add one tablespoon of bran or wheatgerm to prepared breakfast cereals.
- Add dried beans, dried peas, brown rice or lentils to soups and casseroles.
- Thicken soups and casseroles with bran or wholemeal flour.
- Choose wholemeal rolls and sandwiches, fruit salad or fresh fruit when ordering takeaway food.

replaced by food containing more carbohydrate. But Table 9.7 provides some suggestions for further boosting fibre intake.

## IMPLICATIONS

1. Dietary fibre intake (from both soluble and insoluble sources) should be increased to a level greater than 30 grams per day.
2. Increased consumption of fluids may be necessary with extra fibre.
3. Inform clients that they may experience greater flatulence from extra fibre.
4. Select foods with resistant starch as they provide similar benefits to fibre.
5. People with diabetes should choose foods with a low GI to reduce fluctuations in blood glucose.
6. The use of foods high in sugars may need to be limited by some clients.
7. Encourage the consumption of a wide variety of unprocessed plant foods, including fruits, vegetables, wholegrain cereals, legumes, pasta and rice.
8. Clients should be encouraged to eat more wholemeal or wholegrain bread (with low-fat spreads and toppings) per day.
9. Read food labels for starches and fibre.
10. Choose foods labelled to indicate a higher fibre content.

# 10

# Hunger, appetite and eating behaviour

SUMMARY OF MAIN POINTS

- Hunger is a strong *physiological* sensation regulated in the hypothalamus.
- Appetite—physiological, psychological and social—influences eating behaviour.
- Distinguishing between biological hunger and emotional hunger is important.
- Nutrients in food vary in their ability to suppress hunger, and dietary fat has the least effect on decreasing total energy consumption.

In this chapter we go beyond the simple energy value of food and take an in-depth look at another important, but often neglected, aspect of human eating behaviour—hunger and appetite regulation. Hunger is the strong *physiological* sensation which drives us to find and eat food. It has been called a 'biologically useful sensation' because of its obvious survival value. It is part of wider appetite mechanisms which include psychological dimensions.[1]

Our hunger and appetite mechanisms, however, seem to provide little defence against the variety of food and ever-present cues to eat in our modern society.[2] Genetic research is now showing that the feeling of 'fullness' or 'satiety' may be partly genetically determined, such that some people have better 'switch

143

off mechanisms to tell them that they are full. Recent insights into the complexity of the human feeding machine may help us to resolve some old puzzles and lay the basis for a more thorough understanding of eating and obesity.

## HUNGER

Despite our personal familiarity with hunger, it is an extremely complex phenomenon. It is not just an empty stomach that causes that nagging feeling. To simplify things, we need to look at a number of levels of control.

The ultimate decision-maker lies in the brain. The hypothalamus is the part of the brain given the title of 'master control'. Like all good managers, the hypothalamus receives reports from various parts of the body indicating 'fullness' or 'emptiness'. The latter then prompts the drive to eat. Research with flies, which are very simple organisms, shows they have a neural connection from the stomach to the hypothalamus which acts like an eating 'thermostat'. As the stomach becomes distended, a message is sent to the brain to reduce eating. If this connection is severed surgically, the fly no longer has the feedback response and will eat until it literally bursts.[3]

In humans, the connection is much more complicated. The sometimes difficult task is to sort out relevant signals and make wise decisions about food intake.

### Hypothalamic regulation

The function of the hypothalamus is critical for body weight regulation. Research with rats has shown that damage to the

---

MYTH-INFORMATION

*Meal replacement drinks, with added herbs (to make them sound 'natural'), do not contain any 'magic' weight loss formula. They help weight loss in the short term because of reduced energy input. However, they cannot be sustained, and a physiological adjustment generally means they will eventually cause increases in body fatness.*

---

hypothalamus can have serious consequences. Damage to the ventromedial hypothalamus (VMH) is associated with hyperphagia (over-eating), decreased thermogenesis and spontaneous activity, and elevated insulin levels. Obesity is almost an inevitable result. On the other hand, destruction of the lateral hypothalamus, only microns away, is associated with decreased food intake and a reduction in body fat.[4]

These changes are partly influenced by the actions of chemical messengers, called neurotransmitters. Different types of neurotransmitters function to stimulate specific areas of the brain responsible for certain mental states. There are a number of neurotransmitters that can either promote or discourage feeding. For example, *seratonin*, derived from the amino acid *tryptophan*, can reduce food intake and this is now the basis of several appetite-suppressing drugs. Ingestion of carbohydrate results in the release of seratonin which inhibits the further intake of food. Conversely, another neurotransmitter in the brain, *neuropeptide Y*, stimulates food consumption. There are a number of other chemical messengers that either stimulate or inhibit food intake—the strength of specific signals after a preferred food has been eaten may affect that food's desirability for further consumption.

Isolation of a 'satiety' gene, by geneticists working at Rockefeller University in 1994 (see Chapter 16), suggests that genetics may play an important part in hunger. Research carried out over several years has suggested there may be a mechanism coded for by a gene or genes, which 'switches off' hunger signals in the hypothalamus. Scientists have searched for, found, and now synthesised a protein hormone which they have called '*leptin*' (*leptos* is Greek for 'thin') which may result in major advances for drug therapy for obesity—if it lives up to its early promises.

In addition to dealing with neurotransmitter signals and proteins, the hypothalamus integrates a wide variety of messages, from the first smell of food to its metabolic fate as stored energy, by a series of neurotransmitters, hormones and signals from circulating nutrients.

*Physiological signals*—Stomach and intestinal distension are mechanisms for terminating feeding by negative feedback via the nervous system. The release of hormones such as cholecystokinin and the stimulation of special receptors in the gut also provide signals to reduce feeding.

*Nutrient signals*—Circulating glucose, amino acids and fatty acids may also signify that food has entered the body's system and reduce the desire to eat. Low blood sugar levels promote hunger and it is possible that lesser degrees of changes in blood sugar may also influence appetite mechanisms.

*Hormonal signals*—A variety of hormonal changes occur in response to ingested and absorbed nutrients and some of these may influence appetite mechanisms. Insulin is one of the main hormones involved in nutrient metabolism but its role in appetite mechanisms has not been clearly identified.

*Metabolic signals*—The conversion of nutrients into storage tissues may influence appetite mechanisms. For example, the amount of carbohydrate and glycogen stores or fat in adipose tissue may feed back signals to the hypothalamus, giving it important information about the status of the body's energy reserves.[5]

From this wealth of feedback the brain must sort out relevant signals and make decisions about food intake. When hunger is high, an individual's ability to inhibit inappropriate food choices is reduced. Many food companies, especially snack food manufacturers, exploit this by advertising their products on television around meal-times.

## Psychological and social signals

Non-physiological signals can have a profound influence on food choice, quite independent of the physiological signals e.g.:

*Social custom*—This may over-ride physiological hunger. Celebrations held for recreational or spiritual reasons invariably centre around food and drink. In some societies the obligation to eat can go beyond feasting. In the South Pacific in earlier times, for example, women were fattened up with chicken fat to make them more desirable for prospective husbands.[6]

*Time of the day*—Most Western societies tend to have set family breakfast, lunch and dinner times, perhaps reinforced by the school bell. One classic study has shown that the time on the clock may easily over-ride the natural hunger mechanism. When one group of people were kept in a room with a clock running faster than normal, they became hungry and ate their meals before another group kept in a room with a clock operating on normal speed.

*Food availability*—Individuals have specific food preferences. Increasing the number of available food items will increase the probability that all individuals find more of their favourite foods.

Controlled experiments demonstrate that people, like rats, consume larger meals when given multiple foods than when offered a single food (you can do your own research at a buffet restaurant). Whereas in the past, limited food choices may have led to monotony and discouraged intake, this is no longer the case with our vast variety of foods.

*Food palatability*—Palatability is largely determined by the flavour of food—taste, aroma, texture and temperature. Fat is highly palatable due to its creamy texture, and much of the flavour of food comes from volatile fatty acids.

*Other factors*—Restrained eaters, due to their constant dieting vigilance, may have periods of increased appetite, especially when their control or 'willpower' is compromised, such as during periods of stress and grief.[7] This helps explain why some people eat despite not being hungry and also refrain from eating despite being hungry.

### The satiety cascade

The many processes of hunger and appetite regulation have been brought together in the form of the 'satiety cascade'.[8] The schematic representation of the eating process shown in detail in Figure 10.1, provides us with a means of linking the above factors to provide more information about how hunger and appetite work together to regulate eating behaviour.

While this cascade emphasises the physical factors, the psychosocial factors also help to determine both the size of the meal (satiation) and the length of time before we next eat (satiety).

The stages involved in satiation and early and late satiety have been described as *sensory, cognitive, postingestive* and *postabsorptive*. In real life, these stages will overlap and their effects can combine to affect eating behaviour.

*Sensory effects*—are stimulated by the flavour of food. We are not sure how different people react to different sensory factors, but we do know that taste is a stronger predictor of energy consumed from foods than their perceived 'fillingness'.[9] Fast food manufacturers seek to create a 'bliss point' where their foods have maximum sensory desirability.

*Emotional and cognitive effects*—are the eater's feelings and knowledge about the properties and effects of food. Men and women may react differently, for example, in reaction to stress.

**Figure 10.1: The 'satiety cascade'**

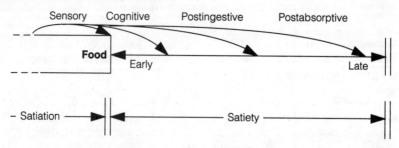

*Source:* Blundell J. et al (1988)[8]

Women are perhaps more likely to react with increased appetite, whereas men may decrease their food intake.

*Postingestive effects*—reflect gastrointestinal signals, i.e. how full the stomach gets, how quickly it empties, the release of hormones to signal 'fullness' and the stimulation of physiochemically specific receptors along the gastrointestinal tract.

*Postabsorptive effects*—include nutrient, hormonal and metabolic signals, plus the possible effects of these on neurotransmitter function. This feedback mechanism probably gives the brain information on the body's energy stores.

## DISTINGUISHING BETWEEN HUNGER AND APPETITE

From a practical perspective, there are two main types of hunger which can be distinguished by the average person. The first is *biological*, or real, hunger. The second is *emotional* hunger, or socially- and psychologically-influenced appetite. Recognition of the distinction is important because this may enable an individual to restrict over-eating in circumstances when it is not warranted, and also provide clues as to when to eat to reduce overwhelming cravings.

*Biological hunger* is where:
• the hunger is genuinely physiological
• the hunger doesn't go away if you wait (e.g. 15 minutes) before eating
• the hunger increases over time
• alternative distractions will not reduce the craving.

In contrast, *emotional hunger* is where:
• the hunger is psychological rather than physiological

- the hunger is likely to go away or decrease in intensity if you wait
- the hunger doesn't increase over time
- alternative distractions can reduce the craving.

One way of personally assessing the level of hunger with a view to decreasing unnecessary eating is to rate hunger on a scale such as that shown in Table 10.1. Experiencing extreme ratings on the scale should be avoided whether going without food (ravenous) or eating too much food (beyond 'full'—feeling ill). When experiencing hunger (ratings below four), a self-assessment of the relative influence of biological and emotional hunger will assist individuals to determine whether they truly have a physiological need to eat or if they are, in fact, finding difficulty in controlling their psychological appetite.

## NUTRITIONAL ASPECTS OF APPETITE CONTROL

The concept of the satiety cascade implies that the effect of any given food will depend on its own unique nutrient composition. This poses a number of questions:

- how do the different nutrients in food contribute to satiation and satiety by suppressing hunger?
- will the suppression of hunger reduce energy intake or cause a compensatory increase at meals eaten later?
- do different nutrients affect fat loss or gain?

Keep in mind that many of our ideas about the nutritional aspects of appetite control come from studies on laboratory rats. These can be far removed from the real world of takeaway pizza, so we need to be cautious when extrapolating these animal findings to humans.

Unlike excess dietary fat intake, which has a clearer relationship to gains in body fat, the various factors that influence appetite

**Table 10.1: A subjective hunger scale**

| | |
|---|---|
| 8 | Beyond 'full'—feeling ill |
| 7 | Very 'full' |
| 6 | Slightly 'full' |
| 5 | Feeling satisfied |
| 4 | No hunger |
| 3 | Slightly hungry |
| 2 | Hungry |
| 1 | Ravenous |

---

**MYTH-INFORMATION**

*Meal replacement biscuits are generally high in energy and fat. They would only work if they could control the intake of food later in the day—and they don't!*

---

may vary greatly between individuals. Let's look at the evidence for different nutrients.

## Fat

A preference for fatty foods may have developed during hunter–gatherer times because high-fat foods were both scarce and probably beneficial for survival.[10] This legacy now counts against us in a world of greater availability of fatty foods with desirable textural qualities like thickness and smoothness.

Does a high-fat meal reduce appetite? Professor Blundell and his colleagues at Leeds University have studied the effects of dietary fat on feeding patterns in humans. They have shown that the most important determinant of the amount of energy consumed in a meal was the macronutrient content of the meal and not the prior level of hunger. For comparison, subjects were required to eat a high-fat dinner one day and then a high-carbohydrate dinner on another day. The results shown in Figure 10.2 indicate that twice as much energy was consumed at the high-fat meal. Surprisingly, the high-energy, high-fat meal did not suppress eating later in the day, nor did it have a significant effect on energy consumed the following day when compared to the lower energy high-carbohydrate meal.[11]

This means that periodic exposure to high-fat meals will lead to over-consumption of energy which is never compensated for later. Fat can also leave a type of 'fat hangover' which causes a person to feel full or bloated, but still with an appetite to eat more. It is useful to learn to recognise this 'hangover' and to realise that it can be avoided (by reducing the fat content of meals). In a practical sense, it is always easy to slip some more fatty food (e.g. chocolate dessert) in at the end of a meal, but this is much less likely to happen with carbohydrate.

## Carbohydrate

The satiety value of carbohydrate is clearly greater than fat,

**Figure 10.2: Energy intake after high-fat and high-carbohydrate foods**

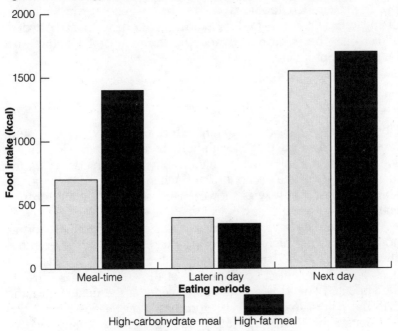

*Source:* Blundell J. et al (1988)[8]

however this varies according to the type of carbohydrate. The properties discussed in Chapter 9, including a low glycaemic index and a high resistant starch or fibre content can all act to boost the satiety value of specific carbohydrate-rich foods.

The relationship between appetite and the commonly reported 'carbohydrate addiction' is less clear. This dietary phenomenon supposedly occurs because of a central imbalance in the metabolism of the neurotransmitter seratonin.[12] The consumption of carbohydrate-rich foods is believed to boost seratonin levels, promote satiety and induce a mood calming effect.

Based on this hypothesis, all carbohydrates should be able to satisfy uncontrollable cravings (a baked potato should do the job just as well as a doughnut). However, this is not the case according to Professor Adam Drewnowski from the University of Michigan. He suggests that it is the 'powerful hedonic synergy' of fat and sugar that forms the basis of food cravings. In an interesting study, he discovered marked differences in food preferences between men and women. When males were asked to list 10 of their favourite foods, they expressed preferences for meat, fish and eggs. Obese women rated ice cream, chocolate, cookies, dough-

151

nuts and pies high on their list. He concluded that whilst men prefer protein-rich foods, women's desires tend toward mixtures of sugar and fat.[13] This finding indicates that the term 'carbohydrate addict' may be a misnomer and the term 'sugar–fat addict' may be more appropriate.

### Fibre

Fibre probably has an important effect on satiety. In one study researchers showed that a high-fibre breakfast, including 20g of soluble and insoluble fibre, significantly suppressed *ad libitum* lunch energy intake 4 hours later when compared with a low fibre breakfast. There was, however, no significant effect on total energy intake for the day.[14]

Other studies have found increased feelings of fullness for 3–4 hours after eating high-fibre breakfast cereals.[15] The highest scores always corresponded to the highest fibre content. Because fibre does not seem to limit consumption at the test meal it seems that the appetite benefits of eating fibre emerge at the next meal rather than the current meal. That is, fibre has a bigger effect on satiety than satiation. However, simply adding fibre supplements to a high-fat diet is not likely to have the same effect as eating a selection of high-fibre foods. This is because the fibre in supplements is not 'bound' to the nutrients in the food consumed.

### Protein

Protein is believed to be the most satiating of all the macronutrients. An intense satiety may last for 2–3 hours after a meal. Therefore if eating occurs during this period, the food intake may be reduced.[16]

The differences in the appetite effects of the above three macronutrients are summarised in Table 10.2. From an appetite perspective, it can be easily seen why the chronic over-consumption of dietary fat occurs with relative ease.

### Alcohol

Light drinkers add alcohol calories to food calories resulting in higher energy intakes than non-drinkers.[17] This is not surprising given that alcohol intake does not produce satiety. In fact, alcohol may stimulate appetite. Alcohol also lowers inhibitions and this

**Table 10.2: Appetite characteristics of macronutrients**

| Factor | Fat | Carbohydrate | Protein |
|---|---|---|---|
| Olfaction | Strong | Weak | Weak |
| Mouth feel | Creamy, smooth | Varies | Limited & varied |
| Flavour | Intense | Less intense | Less intense |
| Effect on satiation | Weak | Strong | Strong |
| Effect on satiety | Weak | Strong | Very strong |

may lead to over-consumption of readily available, high-fat food. Hence, although alcohol *per se* may not result in increased fatness (see Chapter 5), use of alcohol may have this result through its other effects.

This situation is different in heavy drinkers (15–40 per cent of energy intake from alcohol), who appear to burn alcohol inefficiently; in fact, alcoholics who rely on alcohol for most of their calorie intake tend to be thin and malnourished.

## Other food components

### Artificial sweeteners

These have been developed on the premise that sweetness without calories would assist fat loss, but the link appears to be tenuous, at best. Because carbohydrate, including sugar, naturally suppresses appetite, the rationale for artificial sweeteners for fat loss is limited for most people. The biggest users of artificial sweeteners are obese people and research suggests that people who use artificial sweeteners do so to express their fat-loss concerns rather than decrease energy intake (i.e. they may make up for the loss of calories somewhere else).[18] There is some concern that artificial sweeteners increase appetite, but a comprehensive look at all the research on sweeteners by Professor Drewnowski shows there is no evidence that sweetener use *per se* causes increases in food intake by increasing the appetite.[19] The use of artificial sweeteners *in conjunction with other dietary strategies* may be useful in limiting energy intake and there is no substantive evidence to suggest any ill-health effects from use of sweeteners, in moderation.

### Fat substitutes

Dietary fat substitutes have been designed to mimic the sensory properties of fat and enable the production of low-fat foods that can satisfy consumers. There are a number of ways to make a fat substitute. Some are made from carbohydrates and protein, whilst others are derived from other food components (e.g. cellulose), or are completely synthetic compounds. Fat substitutes must be safe to use, must not affect the organoleptic properties of the food and provide some of the attributes of fat.

The biggest question is whether they provide dietary assistance for body fat management? The answer appears to be *yes* when all high-fat foods are substituted for reduced-fat varieties or fat substitutes. If only a portion of high-fat foods (e.g. only ice cream and biscuits) are modified, there is likely to be compensation in the form of extra fat or energy intake at other times in the day.[20] This trend has occurred with low-fat yoghurt consumption, as was mentioned in Chapter 8. Based on current evidence it seems that a complete dietary overhaul to include low-fat options will be most effective for fat loss.

On a practical level, the use of the recently approved (though only in the US) fat substitute *Olestra* has been found to reduce feelings of deprivation associated with low-fat diets, as well as reducing the number of high-fat foods that were considered 'tempting'.[21] Even so, Olestra has serious nutritional implications, as it has also been found to decrease the absorption of anitioxidant carotenoids, vitamin E and other fat-soluble compounds.[22] Oelstra is not yet available outside the US and its potential introduction to other countries will receive fervent opposition from dietitians.

It will be important to monitor a client's use of fat substitutes, artificial sweeteners and reduced-fat foods to see if these dietary modifications are effective.

## Chocolate

This food deserves special mention as it is commonly the typical object of food cravings. There is now some scientific evidence to explain the anecdotal need for a 'chocolate fix'. Chocolate contains phenylethylamine, an addictive substance that affects the brain to produce a pleasure response. This mild 'high' involves the same opiate chemicals or endorphins which respond to some illegal drugs. It is hypothesised that uncontrollable eating binges experienced by some individuals are triggered by an imbalance in the opiate system.[23]

Preliminary experiments which have blocked the action of opiates point to sugar–fat mixtures as the predominant foods of desire. A chocolate addiction may also have something to do with its sensory ('party in your mouth') properties or its frequent use as a special gift or reward.

In line with the belief endorsed throughout this book that for success, lifestyle changes must be those that are enjoyable, there should be no suggestion that chocolate (or any food) be 'banned' from the diet of someone wanting to lose fat. On the contrary, if it is eaten, only the very best (and most expensive) chocolate should be eaten—and savoured—but in small quantities! However, keep in mind that clients who regularly binge on chocolate or other 'bliss point' snacks may require more specialised attention.

---

### MYTH-INFORMATION

*Appetite-control lozenges generally have an anaesthetic ingredient which numbs the tongue and throat. This makes eating uncomfortable. It does not suppress the appetite.*

---

### THE SATIETY INDEX

Researchers at the University of Sydney have recently come up with an interesting new way of rating the satiety of food.[24] Dr Susanne Holt, in the School of Nutrition, asked subjects to rate the satiety or 'feeling of fullness' resulting from eating a number of foods and compared this with a standard measure (in this case white bread). The standard was given a Satiety Index (SI) score of 100. Figure 10.3 shows how a list of common low-fat and high-fat foods compared with bread.

As can be seen, those foods that have the highest SI (i.e. potato and porridge) are also high in starch. Those lowest on the SI (i.e. croissant and cake) are high in fat and are generally those that can be eaten even after a filling meal.

The implications of the SI for fat loss are obvious. Foods with a high SI should be encouraged as they provide a feeling of fullness, reducing the total energy intake. Foods with a low SI should be discouraged because these will only lead to a greater total energy intake. The research on SI is only in its infancy and there is clearly much to be learned in this area which may have relevance to fat loss.

### NUTRITIONAL LIMITATIONS ON FAT LOSS

Adopting life-long healthy eating habits requires a lifestyle fit, with minimum disruption and deprivation. After some experimentation

**Figure 10.3: Satiety index of selected foods**

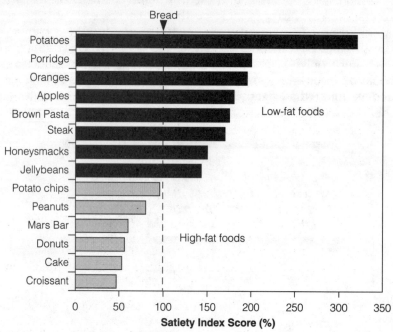

*Source:* Holt et al (1995)[24]

each client will discover what she/he has to do (nutritionally) to control body fat. The key is getting the maximum benefit from minimal change. Each individual will need to set dietary priorities, a process which requires a brief explanation.

Although eating for fat loss requires a reduction in energy intake, counting calories is likely to be counter-productive. It is the source of calories which is important and there is a hierarchy for dietary restriction of specific sources. Fat, with the greatest energy content (9 kcal/g) is a suitable first target for dietary modification. Alcohol has 7 kcal/g and is a secondary consideration. Next on the list is carbohydrates as sugars (4 kcal/g), finally followed by carbohydrate as starch (still 4 kcal/g). If body fat goals are met by targeting fat intake alone, then less emphasis on decreasing other energy sources is required.

If clients cut back on fat, alcohol and sugar and still want to get more off their waistlines, the only thing left is to reduce starchy carbohydrate foods like bread, pasta, rice, potato and corn. This last modification will markedly decrease the volume of food intake, but will challenge hunger and appetite regulation. Severe restrictions in food intake may trigger binges and result in a situation worse than existed initially. This will signal that dietary efforts have been too drastic.

This explanation shows that there is a method for success, and that at some stage the limitations of dietary change will be experienced. Going short on the body's preferred energy fuel (starchy carbohydrates) has its hazards. It is important for clients to be aware of this risk and to put effort into increasing their level of movement. Increasing energy expenditure will allow them to eat more, giving flexibility to their eating program.

## IMPLICATIONS

1. Be aware of the physiological causes of hunger and cravings. This may reduce guilt in clients and increase motivation to combat difficult periods.
2. Tease out factors enhancing appetite such as social custom, food availability and restrained eating, and encourage an awareness of these for modifying eating behaviour.
3. Encourage slow eating to give the body a chance to recognise that feeding is taking place.
4. Graze rather than gorge so as not to risk periods of intense hunger. Snacking every 3–4 hours (using low-fat, sweet foods such as fruit) can promote satiety and reduce possible dietary compensation that may occur at a 5–6 hour time period.
5. Differentiate between biological and emotional hunger and rate levels of hunger to reduce unnecessary over-eating.
6. Wait 15 minutes before eating to see if a craving is physiological or emotional.
7. Reduce availability of high-fat foods. Sensory properties may influence susceptible individuals.
8. Choose high SI foods where possible to maximise satiety, e.g. All Bran, porridge, untoasted muesli, pasta, fruits, beans, lentils, spaghetti and potatoes.
9. Where possible, include high-fibre foods at each meal to help maximise satiety throughout the day.
10. If alcohol is consumed, there should be an awareness of the possible increase in food consumption due to reduced inhibition and possible higher intake of fatty foods.
11. The use of artificial sweeteners or fat substitutes may provide benefits to some individuals but requires individual monitoring.
12. Sustaining a low-fat diet for some time may help to reduce fat preference.
13. Don't 'ban' highly appetising foods like chocolate. Encourage

consumption of only the very best, in small quantities, in order to control intake.

14 Be aware of the nutritional limitations on fat loss and advise clients to avoid food restriction beyond their individual threshold of hunger.

# 11

# Fad diets and dieting for fat loss

SUMMARY OF MAIN POINTS

- Sustainable strategies of eating a low-fat diet and maintaining appropriate activity levels are required for long term management of fat stores.
- Fad diets are not sustainable, exploit the vulnerabilities of the overweight and are counter-productive.
- Criteria can be applied to these diets to assess their validity and sustainability.

Long term management of fat stores requires people to develop sustainable strategies in eating a low-fat diet and maintaining appropriate activity levels. The *ad libitum* approach to low-fat eating has been shown to be the most effective and easiest to follow over the long term. The rationale and techniques for doing this have been discussed in previous chapters. One disadvantage of this approach, however, is that it takes longer for success—even though this is likely to be more sustainable over the long run.[1] Hence, there is still often a desire by many for a 'quick fix'. 'Diets' offer this. Fad diets offer it even more convincingly. The most popular diets promise faster and seemingly effortless ways of losing 'weight', contributing to sporadic, and often counter-productive, efforts in weight management.

## FAD DIETS

Popular diets are usually based on *weight* loss, which over the short term may predominantly reflect changes in body water balance and metabolically active tissue. However, the focus should be on sustainable *fat* loss. Fad diets are those that cause *short term* weight losses, but no long term sustainable effects. Like any fad, they go into and out of fashion according to the media attention paid to them at any particular time. As such, they play on the vulnerabilities of the target group, who regard themselves at fault for the long term failure of the diet.

### MYTH-INFORMATION
*Heat pads and electrical devices, although promoted for fat loss, are banned from advertising as such by the Australian Slimming Advertising Code.*

## CRITERIA FOR ASSESSING FAD DIETS

Assessing diets is a specialised task and there are now publications available which assist in rating diets and diet plans.[2,3]

In the US, the National Council Against Food Fraud[4] has suggested the following criteria as a basis for assessing diet plans:

*If the answer to any of the following is 'yes', the program/diet should be regarded as suspect.*

1. Does it promise or imply a dramatic or rapid weight loss of substantially more than 1–1.5 kilograms per week?
2. Does it promote a diet that is extremely low in energy (kilocalories) without the close supervision of recognised, competent health professionals? As a guide, nutritional adequacy for most micronutrients cannot be met if the daily energy intake is less than 1200 kilocalories.
3. Does it attempt to make consumers dependent upon special products rather than being able to base food choice upon foods that are easily available and part of the usual food supply?
4. Are the 'counsellors' actually salespeople given some in-house training to support the needs of the overfat, and do they have a conflict of interests, given profits are linked to the products they recommend and sell?
5. Do they promote unproven fat loss aids such as human chorionic gonadotrophin, electric muscle-stimulating devices, amino acid

supplements, herbal supplements, spirulina, diuretics, starch blockers, passive exercise, acupuncture, body wraps, glucomannan, enzymes, sweating techniques? . . . the list goes on.

6. Do they claim a special technique for 'breaking down' cellulite?

7. Do they encourage the use of appetite suppressants, either prescribed or 'natural', or the use of bulking agents prior to eating in an attempt to modify appetite and hunger?

8. Do they claim that their product contains a unique ingredient or component, particularly given the increasing interest in herbs, to achieve fat loss? Many of the herbs included in products, especially of the powdered or meal replacement type, are gastrointestinal irritants.

*Conversely, the answers should be 'yes' to the following questions for a reputable program.*

1. Does it provide protein, fat, carbohydrate and fibre in amounts recognised and recommended as part of a health promoting eating pattern?

2. Does it follow the principle of accepted food selection guides (for example, the Dietary Guidelines, Healthy Diet Pyramid or CSIRO 12345+ guide in Australia?)

3. Does it offer variety, in that different foods can be selected each day?

4. Is it an eating plan which could be comfortably used for the rest of the person's life?

5. Does it encourage permanent, realistic lifestyle changes including regular exercise?

6. Do the 'counsellors' fully inform the client about any potential risks of the program or the products being promoted?

## Fad diet models

Most of the fad diets incorporate a strategy that has some potential merit in fat loss, or perpetuate a belief that has existed for many years. These diets pick and select amongst the techniques and package them as the new wonder diet. Almost all fad diets require strict adherence to a plan, which means that people are not learning how to cope with their own environment. Very few use the main principle espoused in this book which is that for a fat loss plan to be successful, it has to be something that can be done comfortably for life.

Some of the characteristic strategies employed by fad diets, which may be useful in a more 'balanced' food intake program, but which are ineffective when used alone are:

**Figure 11.1: A typical fad weight loss 'cure'**

> # Non-Stop Weight Loss
>
> # Thrilling Japanese Super Pill Guarantees Rapid Weight-Loss!
>
> ## *eliminates dieting*

*Monotony:* (e.g. meal replacements, single food groups/items, fasting (with or without juice), 'macrobiotic' diets. These limit the selection of foods in an effort to reduce temptation and often use foods that people believe are 'healthy' or to have special properties that burn fat. Examples are the 'grapefruit diet' and high-protein diets.

*Aversive conditioning:* (e.g. water-drinking diets, grapefruit diets, fibre supplements, meal replacements). These work through two general methods: (a) by either linking an unpleasant task such as being sick prior to eating (particularly if about to 'binge'), or (b) by eating a least-liked/filling food first. Examples are 'bran diets' and the 'water diet'.

*Ritual:* (e.g. single food items, fibre supplements, soup diets, meal replacements, fasting). Rituals may take many forms and have a basis in behavioural therapy. Eating may be delayed by completing a set ritual such as setting the table or by preparing an appetiser of raw vegetables. Food may only be consumed in one place with no other distractions (including conversation!) and food records must be updated prior to eating. Enjoyment does not figure greatly here. Examples are the 'egg diet' and the 'macrobiotic diet'.

*Fillers:* (e.g. water drinking and fibre supplement diets, soup diets, macrobiotic diets, liquid protein diets and fruit diets). This strategy works on the principle that if you fill up on high-fibre foods or water then there will be less hunger for other foods. The difficulty is that nutritious foods may be displaced, contributing to a deficient micronutrient intake. Examples are the 'rice diet' and the 'soup diet'.

*Slowed absorption time:* (e.g. high-carbohydrate diets, rice diets, fibre supplements and macrobiotic diets). Bulky, high-fibre foods that require a lot of chewing (e.g. 32 times each mouthful) are encouraged, as is the consumption of water between bites of food. Other strategies include the putting down of utensils after each bite and encouraging conversation between each mouthful. Examples are the 'bran diet' and the 'spinach diet'.

*Fat restriction:* (e.g. fruit and vegetable diets, high-carbohydrate diets, juice fasts and macrobiotic diets). This method has become one of the keys to fat loss, however, many fad diets using this principle still pose a risk to consumers as they adopt many other unsuitable practices as well, including nutrient inadequacy. Examples include 'fruit only diets' and the 'macrobiotic diet'.

*Moderate sugar intake:* (e.g. solid-meal replacement diets, ice-cream diets, juice fasts). This method includes sugar for its satiety value, but may also include high levels of fat, particularly in some meal replacements. If the emphasis is on carbohydrate-rich foods then the basis would be in the right direction. Examples include the 'Drinking Man's Diet'.

*Food combinations:* (e.g. not eating protein and starch together). This method perpetuates myths that foods rot in the stomach because of effects of bad food combinations on gastric emptying rates and this then contributes to accelerated fat gain. This premise is incorrect on many grounds; first, the foods are generally mixtures of all macronutrients and second, the information on digestive physiology and fat storage is incorrect. Examples are the 'Fit for Life diet' and 'Rotation Diet'.

*Fasting and very low energy diets:* These diets are based on the premise that they rid the body of 'toxins' that stop an individual losing fat and also that all the energy is supplied from the body's tissues, guaranteeing weight loss. An understanding of physiology and of research in fat loss, shows that these are unsound methods that may actually work to increase the fat content of the body.

**Advertising and 'Fad Diets'**

Some typical concepts used in fad diet advertising include:

- '100 per cent guaranteed'
- 'instant' and 'phenomenal results'
- 'x kg weight loss in one month' (usually a lot)
- '100 per cent natural and Dr Recommended'
- 'secret ingredients'
- 'supported by Doctors and Dietitians'
- 'lose inches (cm) while relaxing'
- 'secret of the . . . Aztecs, Incas, Hunzas' (insert an ancient tribe of your choice)

---

MYTH-INFORMATION

*The idea that fasting helps fat loss and 'cleanses toxins' has been clearly disproven. Any weight loss is quickly regained through physiological adaptation and few if any of the minerals lost in sweat are 'toxins'.*

---

**Assessing other diet plans**

The modern focus of eating plans for sustainable fat loss is a decrease in total dietary fat and an increase in the proportion of complex carbohydrates, followed in importance by a decrease in total energy intake. When assessing diet plans, these basic criteria need to be kept in mind. It is also important for health professionals providing advice to those seeking fat loss to know just how this is best achieved and to have an understanding of how popular diet plans manipulate the facts. The following is a review of some general diet plans.

*Total fasting*

Otherwise known as starvation. This is not recommended because of the excessive losses of lean body mass that occur. Many people undertake short-term fasts and actually say that they feel better for it! In the short term, it can contribute to micronutrient deficiencies and in the longer term, contribute to increased body fatness and morbidity. Fasting causes the body to lose water, potassium and sodium (as well as active metabolic tissue) which disturb the homeostasis of the body. Fasting becomes self-defeating as people become lethargic and less active, therefore metabolising less body fat. People eventually stop starving themselves, which can have inherent physiological dangers depending on the severity of the fast. Fasting should be avoided.

### Very low-energy diets

These are often available through clinics, where the diet supervisor (usually someone untrained in nutrition) provides some monitoring designed by a medical practitioner. These diets usually provide a formula feed of less than 800kcal/day, which is less than the usual range needed for the resting metabolic rates of most adults. The physiological effects of these diets are less than for fasting, but still carry risks and require medical supervision. The low-carbohydrate content of the formula stimulates the production of ketones which are thought to be responsible for the appetite suppression experienced. The hunger is intense upon reinstating carbohydrate in the diet. These diets should only be administered to morbidly obese people fulfilling strict selection criteria and within the context of a long term management plan.

### Low-energy diets

These diets aim to provide 800–1200 kcal/day which is substantially lower than the resting metabolic rate of even very lean adults. The associated risks of the diet will decrease as the energy intake increases, but one of the main problems is dealing with hunger on these diets. The use of appropriately advised physical activity programs to support these diets is highly recommended.

When these reduced-calorie diets are based on regularly available foods rather than fortified products, there is a small risk of micronutrient inadequacy. Supplementation may be recommended, which would seem to defeat the purpose of creating a lifelong achievable plan that is nutritionally adequate. The needs of pre-menopausal women for iron and all women for calcium may not be met by these diets.

Many of the commercial weight loss organisations base their programs on this type of diet and include interventions in the form of a client attending a centre, a group meeting in community settings or home-delivered meals. The ready availability of frozen, pre-packaged meals for dieters in the supermarket is an area of concern, as these have little relevance to an overall fat loss strategy and are not concerned with nutritional adequacy.

## Some well known diet plans

Diets in most books and magazines advocate energy restriction. Some, such as 'The Complete F-Plan Diet' and 'The Pritikin Program', are based on credible information, incorporating a high-carbohydrate/fibre, low-fat eating plan, although they tend to be extreme and may be difficult to sustain for a lifetime. Less reasonable but readily available diets that either exclude foods or are based on unsupported claims include:

### 'Rotation Diet'

This diet varies energy intake from 600 to 1500kcal/day over a period of 4 weeks. It then provides for a maintenance dietary intake of 1800kcal/day, which increases the likelihood of micro-nutrient inadequacy. The basic premise of this diet is that by rotating energy intakes for weight loss, a rise in resting metabolic rate is achieved. This is NOT supported by research.

### 'Fit for Life'

Probably one of the most widely talked about diets available, this diet is low in milk, meat, breads and cereals, and very high in fruit and vegetables. Encouraging people to eat more fruit and vegetables is desirable, however the diet is based on unsupported claims that fat is accumulated by improper food combinations. It also misinterprets digestive physiology, particularly gastric empty-ing, and claims that certain macronutrient combinations 'rot' in the stomach and release 'toxins'. These claims are NOT supported by research. Refer to Rosemary Stanton's *The Diet Dilemma* for a more extensive review of this diet.

### The 'Dr Atkins Diet' and 'The Drinking Man's Diet'

These diets are based on carbohydrate restriction. Adequate car-bohydrate is required to maintain blood glucose levels, fluid balance and to spare amino acids from being used as a fuel source. Approximately 100 grams of carbohydrate per day is required to achieve the above and to avoid ketosis. Many examples of low-carbohydrate diets have existed over the years and these diets cause diuresis and loss of fluid weight in the first few days due to glycogen and fluid loss. Protein is catabolised contributing to a further fluid and weight loss. Other side effects apart from dehydration include fatigue, postural hypotension, taste changes, halitosis and altered biochemical parameters. Adequate fluid and carbohydrate intake are two nutritional recommendations that are NOT met by this form of diet.

### The Israeli Army diet

This is an eight-day cyclical diet (four by two days) of apples, cheese, chicken, then salad, that has nothing to do with the Israeli Army. It is low energy, nutritionally inadequate, unsound and boring.

### The Mayo Clinic diet

This has occurred in various forms, all capitalising on the good name of the Mayo Medical Clinic in the United States. One of the many forms of this diet requires the dieter to eat lots of eggs, in the belief that the energy used to digest them is more than the energy provided. The Mayo Clinic has disowned this diet. Other diets have also used this premise that the energy used to digest and utilise a food will be greater than that provided by the food. This is NOT supported by research but has not stopped people creating many diets, including the celery diet and negative calories diet.

### 'The Beverley Hills Diet'

The film stars in Hollywood who gave credence to this diet certainly had no idea of nutrition and neither did its author. It talked of fat-dissolving fruits, and how some other foods were not digested by the body but were trapped as fat. It is a dangerous diet: inadequate, unsound and contrary to any research.

## IMPLICATIONS

Weight loss diets abound, all with the promise of eagerly sought results. If any formularised eating plan is to be used, those working in fat loss need to:

1. Look to scientific research for the basis of claims, and ensure the eating plan is not actually a danger to health.

167

2. Sort through the claims and promises for the actual strategies required.
3. Assess if it requires anything special to make it work, including pills, potions or machines.
4. Assess its consistency with recommended food selection guides and the use of locally available foods.
5. Assess the promised rate of weight loss.
6. Assess the energy level and macronutrient composition and compare this with national recommendations.
7. Ensure that it is nutritionally adequate in micronutrients, and not reliant on supplements.
8. Assess the cost of the plan, particularly for long-term implementation.
9. Ensure that it is sustainable, incorporating commonsense food selection and regular, appropriately chosen physical activity.
10. Refer to an appropriately qualified health professional if unsure.
11. Reject any diet promoting a specific food or drink as a fat 'burner'.
12. Consider only those eating plans which are likely to be adhered to for extended periods without alterations to physical nutrient profiles.
13. Be aware that liquid meal replacement diets without an accompanying activity program should only ever be used for the very obese and with appropriate professional supervision.
14. Discourage dieting in favour of healthy eating plans.
15. Keep in mind that diets of less than 1200kcals per day should not be used except under strict professional supervision and only in cases of extreme and life-threatening obesity.

# VI

# MEDIATORS—FAT/
# ENERGY OUTPUT

# 12

# Physical activity and fat loss

SUMMARY OF MAIN POINTS

- Fat is oxidised under aerobic conditions.
- Optimal fat utilisation in unfit people occurs at a lower exercise intensity compared to fit people.
- Fat utilisation also increases proportionately with exercise duration.
- Hence, low–moderate intensity, long duration activity is most appropriate for fat loss in those likely to require this most.
- Increasing both 'planned' and 'incidental' physical activity is important in any fat loss program.
- In general, weight-bearing physical activities are best for fat loss, except perhaps in the initial stages or for the very obese.

Ask anyone what they think is the best way to lose fat and the two sure answers are 'diet' and 'exercise'. And while diet—or at least a change in eating patterns—is well accepted at the scientific level, it is surprising how little scientific support there is for exercise.[1,2,3] Most scientists working in the area will agree that some form of exercise (or perhaps more appropriately, physical activity) built into an individual's lifestyle, is probably more important than food restriction for long term prevention of fat gain, but there is much less agreement on the benefits of exercise in initial fat loss.

Some researchers have pointed to the relatively small levels of energy expenditure involved in significant levels of exercise. It is typical to find popular diet programs, for example, pointing out that walking a kilometre uses only around 100kcal, which is quickly negated by a glass of beer or small piece of cake. However, the benefits claimed for exercise by its exponents are greater than this. Some forms of exercise have been claimed to increase long term metabolic rate (although this remains controversial) and increase fat oxidation. In addition, exercise is often claimed to be much more psychologically pleasurable than restrictive dieting.

One of the problems in assessing the benefits of exercise in fat loss has been the large individual differences in response to a given exercise load, and the many different types of physical activities that have been used in scientific research. The effect of a certain type of exercise in one group of people, such as young women, doesn't necessarily mean that the same type, intensity and duration of exercise will have the same effect on another group, e.g. fat men.[4] In this chapter, we examine the overall prescription of physical activity for fat loss, taking account of physiological and psychological factors in overfat or obese persons *in general*. This reveals some interesting facts which are not within the commonly accepted paradigm for exercise and weight control, including the controversy about the appropriate intensity of physical activities for optimal fat loss. In Chapter 13, individual differences in prescription are considered and suggestions made about prescribing physical activity for different sub-groups for fat loss. Before doing this, however, it is useful to examine how fat is utilised in the energy system and the implications of this for exercise. This requires some detail which may be skipped over by anyone without the technical background. The practical implications are summed up in the last part of the chapter.

ENERGY SYSTEMS

There are three main energy systems that provide fuel for muscle. Two of these are anaerobic (literally, without oxygen), and the third is aerobic (with air or oxygen). The properties of these three systems are shown in Table 12.1.

The final product used by each of these three systems is the high-energy molecule *adenosine triphosphate* (ATP) which, when split, provides energy for the muscles to contract. For those

**Table 12.1: Characteristics of the three energy systems**

| | Anaerobic System (without $O^2$) | | Aerobic System (with $O_2$) |
|---|---|---|---|
| | Phosphate (ATP-PC) | Lactate | |
| Intensity | Very high (45–100% of maximal effort) | High (45–60% of maximal effort) | Low–moderate (up to 75% maximal effort) |
| Duration | Up to 8–10 seconds | 40–60 seconds | Continuous |
| Fuel | Creatine phosphate | Glucose from carbohydrate only | Carbohydrate and fat |
| By-Products | – | Lactic acid | $CO_2 + H_2O$ |
| Recovery time | 50% in 30 seconds 100% in 2 minutes | 1–2 hours | Continuous recovery |

studying exercise performance, it's the outcomes of these energy systems, particularly muscular contraction, and the types of exercises which improve them, which are important.

For those interested in fat loss, however, it is the fuel use, or *substrate utilisation*, operating within these systems and leading to the end product of ATP, which is most important, because this determines the rate at which energy is utilised and excess fat 'burned up'.

---

MYTH-INFORMATION

*Sit-ups to reduce abdominal fatness will result only in a 'tight' fat waist instead of a 'loose' fat waist. Sit-ups can tone muscle but will have little effect on the subcutaneous fat overlaying this muscle.*

---

The energy systems in relation to exercise have been covered in much more detail elsewhere,[5] and so muscle physiology will only be considered in summary form here. We will then look at the metabolic pathways that provide the options for fuel for muscle. The implications of these for exercise planning for fat loss will be considered in detail. These pathways are complicated and much information is still to be learned from research in this area, but the following will provide an introduction for an understanding of the fat-burning process in humans.

## Substrate utilisation in metabolism

All of the major nutrients—carbohydrate, fat, protein and alcohol—

can ultimately regenerate ATP as needed to fuel the body. However, this occurs through different metabolic pathways. This is shown in schematic format using a currency analogy in Figure 12.1.

Basically, when immediate energy is called for to create movement, especially sudden movement, stored ATP and creatine phosphate (CP) in the muscle are used. Using the money analogy, this could be equated to cash. There's no conversion needed here, and the transaction is quick. Energy is supplied for up to 10 seconds and a period of 1–2 minutes is all that is needed to replenish supplies. The whole process is carried out without oxygen (anaerobically). The type of activity which uses this form of energy is short, sharp bursts of 'power' type activity such as short sprints or weight lifting. Because fat is not immediately implicated in the system, there is little role for this type of exercise in fat burning, at least in the short term.

## Exercise intensity and substrate utilisation

Where a more extended form of physical activity demands more energy, glucose becomes the next most immediate source of energy or 'fuel'. For example, after the first 50–100 metres have been run, the ATP and CP stores have been depleted, but the person is still running and needs more energy. The glucose is broken down in a chain of chemical reactions to form a substance called pyruvate (a process called glycolysis which generates 2 ATPs per glucose molecule along the way). It is then broken down aerobically to $H_2O$ and $CO_2$, generating a further 36 ATPs. If the rate of energy demand is greater than the aerobic system's capacity to handle pyruvate, the anaerobic part of glucose metabolism (glycolysis) supplies the energy needed, and the pyruvate is turned into lactic acid. At high concentrations, lactic acid acts to stop muscles continuing to contract.

It should be noted that lactate salts produced from anaerobic glycolysis are not waste products. Lactates are transported out of the muscle to the liver for conversion to glucose or glycogen and to the cardiac muscle which can use them directly as fuel. *Anaerobic glycolysis* can provide energy for intense exercise up to 45–60 seconds, beyond which it's necessary to use oxygen for further fuel breakdown. If oxygen is present for *aerobic metabolism*, there can be a continual breakdown of glucose until, theoretically at least, this is exhausted. In this case, pyruvate is involved in further energy breakdown through a process called the Krebs cycle, during

**Figure 12.1: Metabolic pathways—a currency analogy**

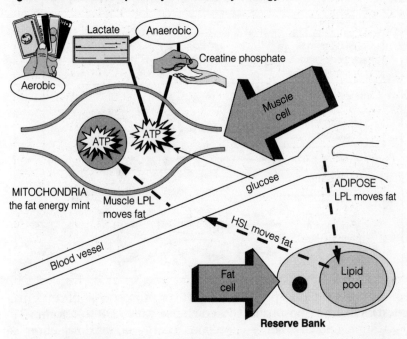

which more ATP is produced (around 36 molecules per glycogen molecule compared to 2 under anaerobic conditions) providing more energy for longer effort. As we have seen in Chapter 3, however, the glucose supplies in the body of a 70kg male only amount to around 450g, or the equivalent of 2250 calories, about a day's energy requirement at rest, and less than would be needed to run a marathon, if glucose was the only fuel source. Hence another source of fuel for physical activity is required.

This is where fat comes into the equation. Fats, in the form of free fatty acids, play little part in the energy equation while there is no oxygen available, because these are only broken down after entering the Krebs cycle where aerobic metabolism is initiated. When oxygen is available, fats take a major role in energy production because each molecule of fat oxidised during this process leads to a production of around 132 ATP molecules, far more than the 36 molecules supplied through slow-aerobic metabolism or the 2 ATP molecules through fast-anaerobic glycolysis.

This process of energy metabolism is shown more accurately (although still in simplified form) in Figure 12.2.

In the top section of Figure 12.2 the mechanism of phosphate reduction and restoration is shown. After stored ATP is reduced

**Figure 12.2: The energy pathways for glucose and fat metabolism**

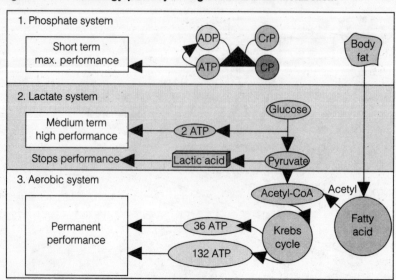

to adenosine diphosphate (ADP) (over 4 seconds of maximal effort), creatine phosphate (CP) combines with ADP to reform ATP + creatine and another 4–6 seconds energy at maximal effort is made available. This process occurs in the cytoplasm of the muscle cell, no oxygen is used and the breakdown of neither fat nor glucose is required. Hence lifting a heavy weight, or an explosion of energy such as in a sprint, burns essentially no fat. In the middle section of Figure 12.2, when a slightly longer term (i.e. 1–2 minutes) of, still intense, muscular contraction is needed, glucose through anaerobic glycolysis is metabolised in the absence of oxygen in the cytoplasm of the cell. Again no fat is involved. When oxygen does become available, such as in the lower third of Figure 12.2, the body uses a mixture of glucose and fat, which is then introduced into the energy cycle through an acetyl group. Fat provides a better option for longer term performance, simply because it is twice as energy dense and there is relatively much more of it than glucose. The key, however, is that oxygen must be present. In other words, the activity must be *aerobic* for fat to be utilised. The extent to which it becomes utilised as part of the energy mix is then dependent on a number of factors, including genetics, state of glycogen stores, the intensity and duration of exercise, the amount of glucose coming from the gut, and the level and type of obesity. Our specific interests here are the exercise parameters that influence fat utilisation and the practical implications of this for general exercise planning.

## FAT MOBILISATION THROUGH EXERCISE

In general, fat is only mobilised significantly *during* aerobic activity. However, because of the energy deficit produced from periods of anaerobic activity (i.e. oxygen debt) and a lack of glucose in the system, fat may be called in to make up this deficit *after* the activity. The limitations, therefore, come in the body's ability to provide oxygen to the working muscles.

There is one further requirement we need to introduce here to understand this fully. Lactic acid is a by-product of anaerobic glycolysis. The build-up of lactic acid develops exponentially with increases in exercise intensity, until a 'threshold' is crossed where extended exercise can no longer be continued (see Figure 12.3). This is called the '*lactate threshold*' or '*anaerobic threshold*' which is the point at which lactic acid production is greater than its rate of removal (although in reality, this is probably not a well defined cut-off point but a phase). As a result, a build up of lactic acid occurs and this is generally considered to be the limiting factor in performance. In practical terms *it is where someone gets so exhausted and 'out of breath' that they have to stop what they are doing and allow the oxygen debt to be repaid.* The anaerobic (lactate) threshold indicates a point above which fat utilisation becomes negligible.

The amount of fat used during exercise therefore becomes dependent on two things:

(1) the total amount of energy used during physical activity
(2) the proportion of this which is below the anaerobic threshold.

Both, in turn, are dependent on the amount and type of exercise carried out, and the aerobic capacity and anaerobic threshold of the individual concerned.

A confusion in the fitness industry often arises in relating these events. It is often argued, for example, that although the proportion of fat utilisation is lower as a result of high intensity exercise, the total amount of energy used is higher, and therefore the *absolute* amount of fat burned for a given individual will be greater at high intensity.[6,7] This is illustrated theoretically in Figure 12.3.

Figure 12.3 compares total energy and fat use at 70 per cent $VO_2$ max versus 50 per cent $VO_2$ max (equivalent to moderate intensity exercise) over a set time period. Fat utilisation at 70 per cent $VO_2$, shown on the right hand side of Figure 12.3, is 40 per cent of energy use compared to 50 per cent at 50 per cent $VO_2$, shown on the left hand side. The higher total energy use at 70

**Figure 12.3: Substrate utilisation with exercise intensity in a trained individual**

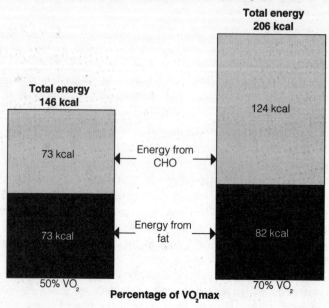

per cent over a 30 minute period (i.e. 206kcal v 146kcal at 50 per cent $VO_2$) means that the absolute amount of fat oxidised is greater at 70 per cent $VO_2$ (i.e. 82kcal of fat energy) than at 50 per cent $VO_2$ (73kcal fat energy). This general view has support from some clinical research,[8] although other work suggests greater fat utilisation at lower intensity.[9,10]

It has thus been suggested that higher intensity exercise (i.e. around 70–80 per cent of $VO_2$ max) will always result in greater *absolute* fat use (even though this type of activity is both de-motivational and potentially dangerous for fat people!) However, this ignores the fact that fat metabolism is related to aerobic fitness and is therefore a graded function of aerobic capacity, which in turn is inversely correlated with body fat levels. A more realistic model than Figure 12.3 is Figure 12.4, which takes account of the heterogeneity of the fat loss response to exercise, particularly between fit and unfit individuals.

Figure 12.4 shows the theoretical differences in oxidative capacity at the same levels of relative exercise intensity for an unfit versus a fit individual. It can be seen from this that as the relative intensity of exercise increases, the ability to oxidise fat decreases at a much greater rate in the unfit than the fit individual. Hence, exercise at low–moderate relative intensities is more likely to provide greater absolute fat utilisation for the fat, unfit person

Figure 12.4: Substrate utilisation with exercise intensity in fit and unfit individuals

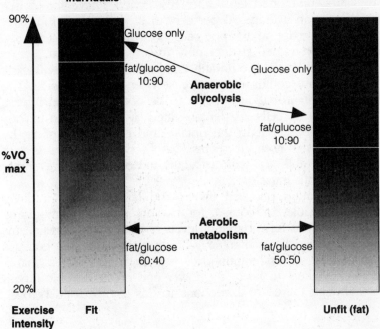

than exercise at a higher intensity. The cut-off point is not definitively known and needs to be more closely researched, but there are indications that exercise at around 40–65 per cent VO$_2$ max is optimal in these people.

This has been demonstrated in research carried out in Denmark[11] in which fit people have on average a 60 per cent greater rate of fat usage during exercise at 60 per cent of their individual maximum effort, than the unfit. Furthermore, the longer the duration of the exercise, the greater the difference becomes. After 3 hours of knee extension work in this study for example, the fit group oxidised up to 85 per cent more fat than the unfit group. A similar result has been demonstrated in individuals before and after improving their fitness through training. Research at Washington University[12] found that before training on an exercise task requiring 64 per cent of VO$_2$ max, the fat utilisation was only 35 per cent of total fuel usage. After 12 weeks of endurance training, fat utilisation rose to 57 per cent of the fuel used on the same absolute task. Another study[13] found that training over 12 weeks increased total fat oxidation by around 41 per cent. A similar effect has even been shown in experiments exercising one trained leg only and comparing the fat utilisation during exercise with that of the other, un-trained leg. Other researchers[14] have found that a trained leg can average 70 per cent of its energy from fat over 2 hours of exercise at 65 per cent of maximal work capacity, whereas its non-trained partner only uses 35 per cent fat.

Again of interest is the finding that fat oxidation plateaus early for the unfit, but continues to increase over time for the fit. The difference in fat utilisation appears to be not so much in release of fat from the fat cells, as demonstrated by the increase in fatty acids in the blood, but in the uptake and combustion of fat by the muscle tissue itself. It seems that fit muscle has a greater supply and is able to 'soak up' intra-muscular fat stores more readily than unfit muscle.

The association between fitness and fatness is not a direct one. It is possible, of course, for two individuals of the same aerobic capacity to have different levels of body fat and this seems to be determined by a number of factors, in particular, genetics and gender. In general though, it's reasonable to suggest that a fat person is likely to be at the lower end of the aerobic fitness scale (although there are exceptions to this as discussed below).

## FITNESS AND FATNESS

The implications of all this are that someone who is unfit is less efficient at using fat in the fuel mix for exercise than someone who is fit, and that this difference increases with the intensity and duration of the exercise. Fat utilisation in an unfit person would therefore only be optimal at an exercise intensity much lower than that required for a fit person—in both absolute and relative terms. This then, gives a totally different outlook to the approach often promoted by the fitness industry based on the 'no pain, no gain' philosophy.

There have also been suggestions that the majority of the energy deficit resulting from physical activity is supplied by fat *after* the activity, or in 'excess post-exercise oxygen consumption' (EPOC), and hence the amount of fat oxidised during the exercise is only part of the story. If this were the case, the total energy use during exercise is again likely to be the biggest factor influencing fat use. However, if we look at this suggestion closely, we see that it is likely to be true first only if the exercise is sustained long enough to significantly deplete glycogen stores, thus diminishing their function as the primary energy source and second, if no carbohydrate is eaten post-exercise, in which case this would take priority as the energy source and fat would once again be 'saved', and deposited into fat stores. This proposal also doesn't explain the increased high rate of re-esterification of fat that occurs in EPOC, particularly in women, probably in defence of their reproductively important energy sources.[15] This is opposed to the approach of re-loading carbohydrate stores for energy after exercise in athletes that is commonly agreed to by exercise physiologists. It does suggest that the issue of type of food intake relating to exercise is more complicated than may first seem.

## DURATION AND INTENSITY OF EXERCISE

RER (respiratory exchange ratio) measures, or the measure of fat and glucose utilisation, need to be looked at for intensity and duration of exercise both for fit and unfit (possibly fat) people, to gain a better appreciation of the appropriate form of exercise for those most likely to be carrying excess fat. Figure 12.5 shows RER scores by exercise intensity. The lower the RER, the greater the reliance on fat.

Figure 12.5 shows that at all levels of intensity, unfit people burn less fat than fit people for a given absolute and relative exercise load. As the intensity increases, this gap becomes even wider (i.e. the difference between x and 2x in figure 12.5). More vigorous exercise obviously burns more total energy in a given time period, but the graph shows that, at least in the unfit, under normal conditions (i.e. no excessively restricted energy intake), higher intensity exercise is likely to be less effective for fat loss. In other words, for an unfit person, the total amount of exercise at this intensity—even if it could be carried out by an unfit person—would not result in substantial fat loss. For a fit person, however, high intensity exercise is associated with fat burning.

Figure 12.6 shows RER by duration of exercise. Here, a similar difference between the fit and the unfit can be seen, suggesting that the longer the effort—at least at moderate intensity—the greater the proportion of fat used in the energy cycle. In the unfit

---

### MYTH-INFORMATION
*'Digital tummy trimmers' are designed to force the abdominal muscles to contract against a tight belt. At best, this may increase some iso-metric muscle strength in the abdominals. It will have no effect on subcutaneous fat.*

---

**Figure 12.5: Substrate utilisation with exercise intensity**

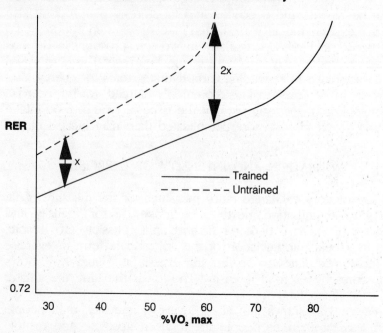

Note: RER is the ratio of oxygen consumed to carbon dioxide produced. Under resting conditions this is referred to as the respiratory quotient (RQ) as discussed in Chapter 4, and is a measure of fat to carbohydrate oxidation. Under dynamic conditions of exercise, more assumptions are needed to infer substrate utilisation ratios. Note, however, sometimes the terms RER and RQ are used interchangeably.

though, some of the research quoted above suggests that this may be true only up to a point, beyond which there is likely to be a decrease in fat utilisation and an increased reliance on glycogen. As fatigue sets in glycolysis plays a more important part, and glucose is thus likely to become more important as an energy source for the unfit, as seen by the upturn in the top curve in Figure 12.6.

These suggestions have been shown in practice in research by Dr David Kelly from the University of Pittsburgh.[10] Kelly exercised obese people over a week for either 50 minutes at 70 per cent of their maximum capacity, or for 70 minutes at 50 per cent of their maximum. Both treatments resulted in exactly the same calorie expenditure. But the RER and total fat oxidation were higher for the longer, less intensely exercised group. Their total fat utilisation was estimated to be 24.5 grams for the 70 minutes, compared to 13.1 grams for the more intensely exercised group. Because fat utilisation is known to decrease in the unfit with

**Figure 12.6: Substrate utilisation with exercise duration**

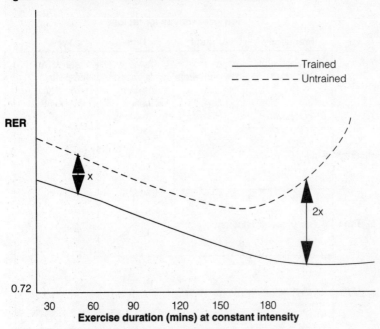

duration of exercise (see Figure 12.6 above), this suggests that for unfit people, fat utilisation would be even greater in the less intense group if the same time period (i.e. 50 minutes) was used for exercise.

All this suggests a change in thinking about the right parameters of exercise for fat loss in unfit (which include most fat) people. The FITT (frequency, intensity, time and type) mnemonic (shown on the left hand side of Figure 12.7) may be appropriate for improvements in fitness, but this needs to be modified for changes in fatness—at least in fat, unfit people. The suggested modifications are shown on the right hand side of Figure 12.7.

As we'll see in Chapter 13, even this model has reservations when it comes to prescribing exercise for specific population sub-groups (women, older people, children etc.). Interestingly though, the new FATT factors shown in Figure 12.7 also agree with the physical activity requirements for wider health gains.[16] Several recent long term studies have shown that high intensity exercise is not necessary for health, or *metabolic* improvements, such as decreased risk of heart disease. Regular, low intensity, long duration activities can be sufficient to provide these improvements. Recently, it has also been shown that in obese people,

**Figure 12.7: Physical activity parameters for fitness and fat loss**

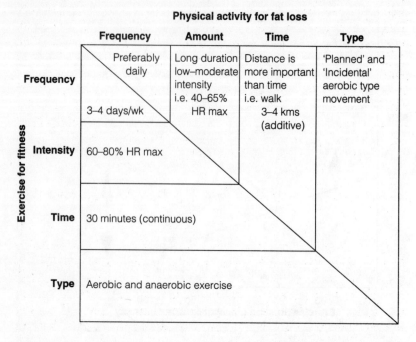

Physical activity for fat loss

|  | Frequency | Amount | Time | Type |
|---|---|---|---|---|
| Frequency | Preferably daily<br><br>3–4 days/wk | Long duration low–moderate intensity i.e. 40–65% HR max | Distance is more important than time i.e. walk 3–4 kms (additive) | 'Planned' and 'Incidental' aerobic type movement |
| Intensity | 60–80% HR max | | | |
| Time | 30 minutes (continuous) | | | |
| Type | Aerobic and anaerobic exercise | | | |

(left axis label: Exercise for fitness)

short (10-minute) bursts of exercise, four times daily, are more effective in fat loss (and even in fitness gained) than continuous (40-minute) bouts. This is primarily because it is easier for obese people to comply with the demands of shorter bouts.[17]

## RISKS OF HIGH INTENSITY EXERCISE

Irrespective of the arguments presented above, there are limitations to the prescription of intensive exercise for overfat people, which make high intensity exercise prescription for fat loss both impractical and irresponsible. Because of the inverse association between body fat and cardiovascular fitness, high intensity activity in people with low cardiovascular efficiency may be potentially dangerous, even fatal. Strenuous exercise is uncomfortable and it may result in overfat people becoming totally disenchanted with physical activity as a fat loss technique. It may also help explain the failure of the fitness industry to attract significant numbers of the almost 1 in 2 people requiring weight control services in Western countries.

A further argument given for high intensity activity is that, given a set period of available time, more vigorous activity provides more 'bang for the buck' in terms of body fat utilisation. If the time is extensive enough to allow for adequate fat utilisation, however, a fat unfit person is unlikely to be able to complete an exercise session at a high (e.g. 70–80 per cent $VO_2$) level of intensity. Even if it were possible, Figure 12.6 suggests a diminishing effectiveness of response in relation to fat utilisation with longer duration which would defeat the purpose of the exercise. Because exercise at such a high intensity may also be uncomfortable for such a person, he or she is not likely to want to do it on a regular basis, as is necessary for optimal fat loss.

## PHYSICAL ACTIVITY AND 'INCIDENTAL' EXERCISE

One of the problems in designing physical activity for the overfat is the negative connotations of the term 'exercise'. This is probably to do with the association of exercise with high intensity activity. A greater emphasis on low–moderate level activity, and a shift from the notion of exercise as 'extra-curricular' to lifestyle changes in activity patterns suggests that a term such as physical activity might be more appropriate. There are two forms of this that are relevant:

- *'Planned'* physical activity, such as walking, swimming or some other form of aerobic activity carried out regularly, often as a part of recreation.
- *'Incidental'* physical activity, such as walking up stairs instead of using an elevator, walking instead of driving, or even not using effort-saving devices such as cordless telephones or remote controls for television sets.

Planned physical activity is necessary to compensate for the decrease in daily energy use resulting from changes in work and daily living conditions in most modern societies. Weight-bearing activities such as walking are likely to be the most effective because of the greater energy use. However, in the first instance, non-weight-bearing activities such as swimming, which are thought to be generally less effective in fat loss, may be more able to be carried out and therefore less de-motivational. A summary of the advantages and disadvantages of some of the different forms of planned exercise for fat loss is given at the end of this chapter.

Incidental activity is designed to counter reductions in spontaneous physical activity that occur in technically advanced societies. It is this which may be of most importance, and may initially even be the only exercise prescription for obese, in contrast to overfat individuals, because of the discomforting and de-motivational aspects of more vigorous forms of activity. As body mass decreases and planned physical activity becomes more comfortable, different forms of planned activities can be introduced.

## ACTIVITY AND FAT LEVELS

Obviously, all of this is good news for the fat, unfit person wanting to decrease body fatness. Long duration, low intensity regular exercise, such as walking, is obviously less painful and more rewarding than that type of exercise which most fat people regard as masochism. It is also more able to be built into a person's daily life and become part of a total lifestyle program which is vital for long term fat loss maintenance. The low intensity–long duration approach therefore would be welcomed by the unfit. However, it does signal a change in the traditional approach to dealing with overfatness through commercial health and fitness centres. Many of these centre around providing an institutionalised service of 30–40 minutes daily, 3–4 days a week, based on the standard FITT model for improvements in fitness. Little attention is given to other aspects of spontaneous physical activity, or indeed, activity patterns outside the gymnasium setting.

The low intensity approach suggests that where fat loss is the goal, the required change is to the individual's lifestyle pattern of activity, including both 'planned' and 'incidental' activity. The role of the instructor in this framework should be one of *empowering* the individual to be able to incorporate this type of physical activity into their lifestyle. The mode of instruction required therefore is *reflective*, i.e. providing advice to fit the client's perceived needs, rather than *directive*, i.e. providing instruction to fit a pre-set formula to the client.

## DIFFERENT TYPES OF EXERCISE AND FAT LOSS

Although it is not possible to list all the different forms of physical activity here, the advantages of some of the major activities for fat loss are discussed below and in Table 12.2.

## Aerobics

Aerobics, or exercise to music classes are popular, particularly amongst females, because of their social involvement, safety and the support of numbers. Some modern aerobics classes now cater for the body image concerns of big people by insisting on big T-shirts, floppy clothes and no body-hugging leotards (even on instructors). In line with the previous recommendations, aerobics classes should be of only moderate intensity. This gives rise to difficulties in gauging a standard intensity for all participants. Because each person has a different level of fitness, some may be working anaerobically, while others are working well within their means.

Duration and frequency of the activity are also important. The longer and more often classes are taken, the more benefit is likely. But this should not be seen as providing enough physical activity by itself. For many people, particularly the elderly, participating in an organised aerobics class can often result in a reduction in other forms of spontaneous physical activity which may have been done during the rest of the day. Total net increase in energy expenditure may actually be less than before aerobics classes were undertaken. It is important therefore for the fat loss leader to monitor all forms of physical activity, not just that which occurs in organised classes.

## Swimming

Swimming, or exercise in an aquatic environment, is usually one of the first exercises on the list of those recommended for fitness and fat loss. But while it may be good (if used properly) for fitness, there are growing reasons why it is less effective than other forms of weight-bearing exercise for reducing fatness:

- Because body weight is supported, there's less energy required to move while floating in water.
- Because fat floats, the fatter an individual, the less energy is required to stay afloat and move in water (this helps explain why swimming is even less effective as a fat loss technique for women with their higher proportion of body fat).
- The rate of energy expenditure in water is totally dependent on the level of efficiency of the swimmer. A very bad swimmer will burn more energy than a very good one (often produced anaerobically). A good swimmer can also bob along at a rate which has minimal energy requirements.

- Maintenance of core body temperature through heat loss during and after swimming is much easier than during land-based activities. Therefore energy is not required to return the body to normal core temperature.
- A lower centre of gravity in females helps them float better and therefore use less energy than men in water.

This is not to deny some benefits of swimming, in particular the more vigorous forms of 'aquarobics'. Swimming can also be useful for very big people at the beginning of a fat loss program because of the difficulty and pain involved in weight-bearing exercise. The principal benefits however will be in fitness gains for high intensity activity rather than losses in fatness relative to other weight-bearing exercises such as walking.

The main recommendation for swimming then would be very early in a program for a very fat person, to assist initial body mass loss to the point where weight-bearing exercise can be used. Because many big people also have damaged joints, such as ankles and knees, swimming or aquarobics can provide an alternative form of activity. Aquarobics, or exercises in water, may be more effective than swimming because of the resistance provided by water to muscular contractions. Still, this is likely to be less effective than weight-bearing physical activity such as walking and therefore should be used sparingly if the client can, and is motivated, to walk.

### Cycling

As with swimming, cycling is a weight-supported, or non-weight-bearing activity, and therefore of less absolute benefit in fat loss than the non-weight-supportive physical activities. However, again it can have value in the early stages of a program to enable someone to reduce enough fat to carry out other weight-bearing exercise.

### Jogging

Jogging is one of the most effective fat loss physical activities available, but ironically, it is not suited for big or overfat people. It can be quite painful and de-motivating for anyone to carry a large body mass over a distance at speed. It can also be relatively dangerous, not just for the extra pressure put on the cardiovascular system, but because of the possibility of weak joints in the hips, knees and ankles.

**Table 12.2: Ratings of different exercises for fat loss**

*Advantages and disadvantages of different types of exercise for fat loss*

| Exercise | Advantages | Disadvantages |
|---|---|---|
| Walking | Comfortable; convenient; non-weight supportive and therefore high energy use | Not good for knee, ankle, foot injuries; may be difficult in some areas |
| Jogging | Takes less time; can be addictive, good to do with friends | Can be uncomfortable; dangerous for overweight; can cause injury; too hard |
| Swimming | Comfortable; few injuries; good for very overweight because weight is supported; good in summer. (Not quite as good for women as their higher fat level makes them more buoyant so they don't expend quite as much energy.) | Doesn't burn as much energy (because weight is supported); can be taken too easily; cold in winter; sometimes inconvenient. |
| Cycling | Enjoyable; comfortable (because weight is supported) for the very overweight; can be done at different intensities | Not as good for fat burning as non-weight supportive; can hurt knee, hip problems. |
| Tennis/golf | Enjoyable; social; not too energetic | Lack of continuity—stop-start; can be too easy (e.g. doubles tennis) |
| Aerobics | Enjoyable; social; high rate of energy use; muscle tone as well as fat loss | Requires some coordination; needs good instructor; can be too hard (and dangerous) for the very overweight. |
| Skipping | Convenient; high rate of energy use | Boring; can cause leg injury; needs coordination; difficult to carry out for long enough. |
| Squash | High rate of energy use; enjoyable | Dangerous for the overweight; can cause back injury; too vigorous—recommended only for those who are fit and not overweight, not recommended for fat loss |
| Rowing | Good for those with lower body injury; can be portable (rowing machine) | Can be boring. Potentially dangerous for those with lower back problems |

Many men, who lose significant body fat, are then often motivated to jog and this should obviously not be discouraged. It is important to make clear, however, that jogging is not necessary for fat loss, as many people think. The 'no pain, no gain' philosophy may be true for the elite athlete, but it has no relevance for very unfit fat individuals.

## Walking

For most people, walking represents the single most natural, easiest and convenient form of fat loss physical activity. Because it can be carried out at low–moderate intensity over long durations and with low impact, it presents few injury problems or health risks. Walking does not have to be brisk, but most importantly, it should be carried out over a set distance, preferably equating to 3–4 km per day. It can also be increased as part of 'incidental' activity, such as walking up stairs, not using transport, etc. Hence, in the vast majority of cases where injury is not a limiting factor, walking is perhaps the best form of 'planned' physical activity for fat loss.

## IMPLICATIONS

1. Physical activity should be seen as an integral part of any prescription for fat loss except where this may be contra-indicated or is difficult because of injury or other problems.
2. Physical activity should be seen as vital to the long term maintenance of fat loss.
3. The primary recommended form of physical activity for fat loss and long term maintenance of fat loss is long, low to medium intensity, gentle continuous aerobic exercise.
4. The appropriate level of intensity of physical activity for fat loss with optimal safety in someone who is fat and unfit is 40–60 per cent $VO_2$ max.
5. Intensity of physical activity may increase with increasing fat loss and fitness, although this should be prescribed by a relevant medical or exercise specialist.
6. Physical activity prescription in the initial stages of a program is perhaps best based on distance covered in the case of walking, cycling, swimming, etc. With increasing fitness, heart rate and then perceived rate of exertion (PRE) can be used to determine the intensity of physical activity.
7. The frequency with which 'planned' activity needs to be carried out for significant fat loss is daily, or at least 6 days a week.
8. Duration of planned physical activity will affect total calorie use as well as substrate utilisation and therefore no upper limit on duration at low intensity needs to be imposed. Upper limits would be determined by the level of comfort of the individual, as well as limiting medical and physical factors.
9. Non-weight-bearing activities such as cycling, swimming or rowing should be given less support in fat loss programs, except where patients may need this initially for comfort or motivation.
10. Anaerobic activity should never be prescribed for fat loss,

particularly in cases where fitness levels and medical contra-indications are unknown.

11. As well as planned physical activity, 'incidental' activity should be encouraged at other times during the day; this may include walking stairs, walking instead of driving, not using modern technological devices such as remote control units for TVs, etc.

12. Special care should be taken to ensure that clients involved in planned physical activity programs do not decrease their level of spontaneous physical activity at other times during the day as a result of this.

13. Appropriate basic stretching techniques need to be taught to overfat patients to accompany planned aerobic physical activity routines.

14. Variety in physical activity routines is recommended to maintain motivation and ensure a slower rate of energy adaptation to a single exercise form.

15. Special problems of big people—such as chapped thighs caused by walking—should be recognised and accommodated for by appropriate recommendations (e.g. such as the wearing of lycra shorts in the case of chapped thighs).

16. It may be necessary to allow time for physical adaptations to introduced forms of physical activity, such as sore knees, provided these problems do not get worse. Referral to appropriate professionals is necessary if problems persist.

17. Where planned physical activity is not possible as part of a fat loss prescription, more attention needs to be given to the control of amount and type of energy input.

# 13

# Individualised movement prescription for fat loss

## SUMMARY OF MAIN POINTS

- There is a variety of factors which influence the fat loss response to exercise:
  Fixed (age, gender, genetics, race) or variable (climate, diet, degree of obesity, fitness level).
- Exercise parameters (frequency, amount, time and type) can also alter the fat loss response within this range of influencing factors.
- There are arguments for and against resistance training for fat loss, however resistance training for fat loss probably has limited value relative to aerobic exercise.

The general indications for physical activity for fat loss were discussed in Chapter 12. However, it is becoming clear that general prescriptions, while necessary, are insufficient alone as there is a variety of different responses to exercise within individuals and groups of individuals.[1] One main influencing factor discussed previously is gender, with females having a lower fat loss response to exercise than males. There are a variety of other factors which can also significantly influence prescriptions for exercise for fat loss. These can be divided into 'fixed' and 'variable' factors. A third influencing factor, which has been covered in Chapter 12, is differences in prescribed exercise parameters. All these influencing factors are shown schematically in Figure 13.1.

**Figure 13.1: Factors influencing the fat loss response to exercise**

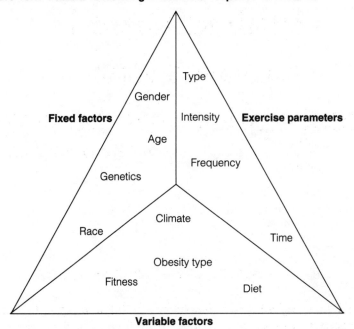

There is a general need for more physical activity in anyone needing to reduce body fat, but the frequency, amount, time and type of activity can vary according to fixed and variable factors appropriate to the individual. While there is no strict science associated with this type of individual prescription at the moment, there are certain guidelines which can assist those working in the area in preparing individualised prescription.

## FIXED FACTORS

A list of fixed factors influencing the fat loss response to exercise and the direction of this influence is shown in Table 13.1. Some of these have been discussed in Chapter 12, so only their relative influence is considered here. Exercise parameters influencing these factors were also discussed in Chapter 12.

### Age

Age differences are most obvious at four different stages—childhood, adolescence, middle age and elderly—but age also interacts

**Table 13.1: Fixed factors influencing the fat loss response to exercise**

| | Main differences in effects | Possible mechanisms influencing |
|---|---|---|
| Age | • Exercise response decreases with age | —metabolic rate<br>—SPA<br>—fat distribution |
| | • Interactions with gender, $VO_2$ level and intensity | —fat oxidation<br>—β receptor sensitivity |
| | • Varied responses to different types of exercise | —associated medical conditions<br>—body composition |
| Gender | • Reduced female response at each level of FATT | —body composition and metabolic rate |
| | • Greater fat conservation in females | —fat type and distribution<br>—biomechanics<br>—hormonal environment<br>—oral contraceptive use |
| Genetics | • Wide individual and familial variation in response to exercise | —body composition and BMR<br>—thermogenesis<br>—fatty food preference<br>—fat oxidation<br>—$VO_2$; SPA differences |
| Race | • Unclear | —fat distribution and body shape<br>—muscle fibre type |

with gender and other variables in influencing the effects of exercise for fat loss. There are big differences between childhood and early adolescence and early and late adulthood in a range of factors which have relevance for fat loss.[2] Metabolic rate, for example, is much higher in childhood and is known to decrease at the rate of around 2 per cent per decade after age 20. This means that by age 70, the body is burning about 10 per cent less energy at rest than it was at age 20, largely due to changes in the fat:lean mass ratio. When this is coupled with a decrease in 'spontaneous physical activity' (SPA), a decrease in the sensitivity of β receptors on the fat cell surface modifying substrate utilisation, changes in body fat distribution and muscle content, and changes in thermogenesis, all favouring a higher fat metabolism in the young, the extra difficulty older people have in maintaining a low level of body fat is more understandable.

Decreases in aerobic capacity and muscle strength suggest that if fat losses are to be gained through physical activity in the older age groups, attention will need to be paid to the total amount of exercise (at a low–moderate intensity) and the level of incidental and spontaneous activity. Maintenance of muscle mass through resistance training may also be important in maintaining metabolic rate which is thought to be reduced due to the atrophy of type II muscle fibres with ageing.

## Gender

There are major differences between males and females in fat loss responses to exercise.[3] Female fat cells are predominantly less lipolytic than those stored around the abdomen of males, and are hence less responsive to exercise. Most researchers now agree that this has a biological function in providing females with an energy reserve for reproduction. There is some suggestion that female gluteal-type fat cells may even be resistant to some types of activity, such as high intensity exercise in younger, pre-menopausal women. Studies carried out at McMaster University in Canada have also shown that, unlike males, female athletes seem to be less effective in 'carbohydrate loading' for long endurance events such as the marathon.[4] (Carbohydrate loading is a technique whereby large amounts of carbohydrate are eaten 3–4 days before an event in order to 'fill' the glycogen reserves which supply immediate energy for the event. This suggests the capacity for glycogen storage is decreased in females and they prefer to use carbohydrate for immediate energy rather than storage.)

Differences in the hormonal environment and body composition lead to a greater fat loss response to a set exercise load in men, and a guaranteed response to almost any form of exercise in younger men. Biomechanical differences and the higher proportion of body fat in women make them more efficient at some forms of exercise, thus using significantly less energy than men for a set exercise stimulus. It has been estimated, for example, that an average-sized woman will use approximately 40 per cent less energy than an averaged-sized man in walking an equivalent distance.[5] Swimming involves an even greater energy differential between genders because of the higher proportion of body fat and the lower centre of gravity in females (enabling them to float more effectively and maintain a more efficient body position). Research at Leeds University in England suggests that females may also eat more after exercise than men, thus making up for the extra energy used during the activity.[6]

All of this has led Dr Gilbert Gleim, a US exercise scientist, to conclude that: '. . . as an isolated weight loss modality . . . exercise should not be counted on to produce desired weight reductions (in women) unless the woman is committed to many hours of exercise a day'.[7]

Exercise prescriptions then need to take account of the greater lipolytic resistance which occurs with reduced energy balance, greater compensatory eating and the reduced muscular response to resistance training. All of this suggests a need for a significantly greater total amount of exercise in females in order to achieve the same fat loss benefits from exercise as a man. On the more positive side, any amount of exercise in women (as well as men) has been shown to improve health profiles such as blood pressure, cholesterol, blood sugars and feelings of wellbeing, even if it doesn't have a major impact on body fat.[8] Older females, with a higher proportion of upper body fat, might be expected to respond more like a man, at least in the reduction of their upper body fat to a given exercise load.

## Genetics

Where there is good reason to suspect a genetic influence on obesity, it is reasonable to suspect that the fat loss response to exercise will be blunted in comparison with the non-obese. Genetic influences probably mean a reduced level of fat utilisation at a given exercise intensity meaning that a greater total amount, and greater attention to the type of energy intake, is required.

---

### MYTH-INFORMATION
*It is often assumed that males and females should lose fat at the same rate through physical activity. This is not so. Exercise appears to be not as effective for fat loss in most women as it is in men.*

---

## Race

Although not yet widely studied, differences in body fat distribution, muscle fibre type, and fat oxidation rates between different ethnic and racial groups could be expected to have an impact on exercise effects between groups. For example, the higher level of glycolytic 'fast twitch' muscle fibre in negroid people and American Indians, which is known to be associated with higher levels of body fatness, could influence the exercise parameters required for optimal fat loss in these racial groups, although the most appropriate approaches are not yet known. Until more research confirms these proposals, the general principle of increased energy expenditure for fat loss is all that can be recommended.

## VARIABLE FACTORS

As well as the unalterable, or fixed factors affecting the fat loss response to exercise, there are a variety of variable factors which can have an effect. Some of these are listed in Table 13.2. The list is not exhaustive, but can give an indication of the complexity of the issue.

### Climate

The effects of cold on the fat loss response to exercise have been studied extensively and have been reviewed by Professor Roy Shephard of Toronto University in Canada.[9] Basically results show that repeated and prolonged moderate exercise in a cold environment creates a greater energy deficit than in a warm environment. Shephard's group demonstrated this with Canadian soldiers on

**Table 13.2: Variable factors influencing the fat loss response to exercise**

| Variable | Main differences in effects | Possible mechanisms influencing |
|---|---|---|
| Climate | • Response greater in cold<br>• Cold effect blunted in females<br>• Clothing effects | —core temperature<br>—shivering thermogenesis<br>—intramuscular glycogen<br>—fat mobilisation<br>—catecholamine sensitivity (females)<br>—metabolic rate |
| Diet | • Fat after exercise can reduce effects<br>• CHO preload immediately prior to exercise decreases lipolysis | —sparing of depot fat<br>—fat and glycogen mobilisation<br>—biochemical energy costs of metabolic assimilation |
| Obesity level and type | • Increased fat loss in obese (although metabolic response may be similar)<br>• Upper body fat responds better to exercise | —aerobic capacity<br>—intramuscular fat uptake<br>—dietary compensation<br>—EPOC<br>—β cell sensitivity<br>—muscle type ratio: FT:ST |
| Aerobic capacity | • Fit muscles more efficient 'fat burners'<br>• Fit women use more fat in endurance exercise than unfit | —oxidative capacity<br>—intramuscular fat use<br>—lactate thresholds<br>—lipolytic sensitivity<br>—fat mobilisation<br>—body composition BMR<br>—muscle fibre type |

Notes: CHO = carbohydrate
EPOC = Excess post-exercise oxygen consumption
FT = Fast twitch muscle fibre
ST = Slow twitch muscle fibre
BMR = Basal metabolic rate

manoeuvres in the Arctic. The fat loss of these men was compared with that of soldiers in mainland Canada in the summer, whilst on an identical dietary and exercise regime.

Explanations for the extra effects of the cold include an altered sensitivity of catecholamine receptors, and increased thermogenesis through shivering. Endurance activity in the cold appears to have specific fat loss benefits, although this effect seems to be less well developed in men than in women. Exercising in the Arctic is obviously the extreme situation, but it probably carries some lessons for fat loss in extreme conditions. Exercise in the cold may give added advantages in therapy for obesity, provided vigorous exercise is not attempted with cold muscles.

Conversely, over-heating by rugging up with warm clothing while exercising, as is often done in an attempt to 'sweat off' fat, may be counter-productive for fat loss. The loss of sweat may result in some weight loss but much of it will be fluid loss.

The body maintains an optimal core temperature of around 37.5°C. In a hot environment, the body has to work to prevent its core temperature from rising. However, the human system for cooling (i.e. sweating) is passive and costs little extra energy and there is also a natural decrease in energy use to allow dissipation of heat. For this reason, techniques of over-heating (i.e. such as saunas and steam baths) are likely to have little long term effect on body mass other than a decrease in body weight through loss of water from sweating.

MYTH-INFORMATION

*It is usually believed that heat treatments are better for fat loss than cold. However, it takes less energy for the body to passively cool itself than it does to maintain body heat. Theoretically then, a freezer would be a better fat loss treatment than a sauna bath.*

## Diet

Individuals on a high-fat diet have been shown to lose less fat in response to exercise than those on a high-carbohydrate diet.[10] High intakes of dietary fat lead to a greater energy surplus which is then stored in depot fat cells, while blood fats and glycogen are utilised for energy. The benefits of exercise are thus at least partially negated by the effects of excess energy in the form of fat. Yet while this is known, it is often difficult to verify.

Recent research using radioactive isotopes has shown that people under-estimate the amount of energy consumed in their diet by around 30 per cent, and over-estimate the amount of exercise they carry out by about 40 per cent.[11] The under-estimate of food intake is reportedly higher in women than in men and there are indications that women may unconsciously eat more after exercise, whether as a means of defence against fat loss or a reward for having carried out exercise. Particular attention therefore needs to be paid not only to the fat content of the diet as a whole, but to the compensatory energy intake following exercise in some women. It's not clear whether different types of exercise have different effects on this level of compensatory eating.

## Degree of obesity

There are a number of physiological factors—e.g. the ability to oxidise fat in response to exercise, and different muscle fibre types[12]—which distinguish the obese from the merely overfat, or the lean. These are also known to affect the fat loss response to exercise. Due to physiological factors that have either caused or resulted from obesity and which are as yet largely unknown, those prone to weight gain may have a greater craving for fatty foods after exercise and may store fat more readily than those not disposed to overfatness.[13]

Exercise responses can also be quite different. Because of the lower levels of aerobic capacity and different rates of substrate utilisation in the more obese, long duration activity and increased 'incidental' exercise at a much lower intensity than is used for the leaner and more fit is recommended for optimal fat burning. There is a case for regarding the morbidly obese as a different population to normal and overfat people in their responses to exercise. The physiological changes that occur with this type of obesity are most likely to be genetically based or associated with long term obesity, and this may provide clues as to the type of exercise and dietary prescription required for optimal fat losses in the future.

### AEROBIC CAPACITY

Aerobic capacity is known to confer definite advantages on the fat loss effects of exercise.[14] The ability to exercise longer at higher levels of aerobic capacity results in an increased rate and earlier onset of fat oxidation, an improved ability of muscle tissue to utilise fat preferentially as an energy source, higher levels of intramuscular fat storage and improved psychological benefits.

## SUMMARY OF PRESCRIPTION NEEDS

There are few specific exercise prescriptions for heterogeneous groups that can be scientifically supported at the moment, but those with most promise appear to be the following:

- long duration, low intensity exercise for pre-menopausal women
- any form of physical activity (high or low intensity) for younger men
- increased resistance training for seniors
- walking is a simple, low cost, moderate intensity activity easily incorporated into lifestyle
- a greater emphasis on dietary change rather than exercise in the initial stages for the obese
- emphasis on small, additive increases in daily physical activity in the obese
- non-weight-bearing exercise (e.g. aquarobics, cycling) in the initial stages for the very overfat
- increased emphasis on SPA and 'incidental' activity with older people
- shorter cumulative bouts of aerobic activity for the unfit.

A summary of hypothesised prescription parameters for some overfat groupings is shown in Table 13.3. Many of these suggestions are tentative and are proposed here as a model for further testing. They are likely to provide a more focused approach to prescription, however, than dealing with all cases of overfatness and obesity as homogeneous.

## WEIGHT TRAINING OR NOT?

Currently there is controversy in health circles about whether weight-training or resistance training (RT) has benefits for fat loss and fat loss maintenance, either independently, or over and above that which may be achieved through aerobic exercise. There are arguments for and against the use of weight training for fat loss as summarised in Table 13.4.

**Table 13.3: Proposed individual exercise prescription for heterogeneous groups**

| Group | Frequency | Amount | Time | Type | Other |
|---|---|---|---|---|---|
| Android shaped males (non-obese)*** | 3–4 days/wk | low/med/high (40–95% $VO_2$) Depends on fitness | 30–40 mins/additive | An/aerobic; non-wt-bearing OK; sport; physical activity | Reduce dietary fat; increase fibre |
| Older males (non-obese)** | 4–6 days/wk | low/med (40–65% $VO_2$) | 40–60 mins or distance of 3–4km walking | Aerobic; weights | Reduce dietary fat; watch for SPA |
| Post-menopausal females (non-obese)* | 6–7 days/wk | low/med (40–65% $VO_2$) | long (1hr +) preferably continuous | Aerobic; weights; non-wt-bearing (e.g. swimming) | Reduce energy intake; watch for SPA |
| Pre-menopausal females (non-obese, unfit)* gynoid male | 7 days | low (40–60% $VO_2$) | long (1hr +) preferably continuous | Aerobic; non-wt-bearing; + 'incidental' ex. | Reduce energy intake (but not <1200–1400kcals) |
| Pre-menopausal females (fit)* | 6–7 days | med/high + low (40–85% $VO_2$) | long (but less than above) i.e. vigorous + extra | An/aerobic; weights; + 'incidental'; wt-bearing | Reduce energy intake (but not <1200 – 1400kcals) |
| Obese (males and females)* | 7 days | very low/low (30–50% $VO_2$) | additive, as comfort permits | 'Incidental' then non-wt-bearing short periods (e.g. cycling) | Diet initially; 'movement' (not 'exercise') for maintenance |
| Children** | 7 days | low/med | additive; reduce sedentary periods | 'Play'; challenge | Make physical activity enjoyable through play |

*Note:* Evidence on effects of exercise on fat loss in this group:
*** well supported
** reasonably well supported
* not well supported

**Table 13.4: Arguments for and against the use of resistance training in fat loss**

| Arguments for | Arguments against |
|---|---|
| • Muscle mass and hence RMR can be maintained | • Resistance training uses less energy than aerobic activity |
| • Upper body muscle mass can be lost through lower body aerobic exercise | • Fat oxidation is greater during aerobic exercise |
| • Up to 25 per cent of weight loss following dieting could be muscle | • Time could be better spent working aerobically |
| • Adds variety and increases motivation | • Resistance training is psychologically difficult for the overfat |
| • Best for maximum fat loss gains in the fit | • Discomfort may turn clients off other exercise |
| • May be good 'second stage' treatment after some fat loss | • Muscle growth is more difficult with age |
| • Could be especially useful in the elderly because of declining muscle mass | • Big people tend to want decreases in size, not maintenance or increase |
| • Improved joint stability | |

Resistance training is a standard form of fitness training in most commercial fitness centres. Yet it is a mode of exercise that has not been extensively studied in conjunction with fat loss. From a commercial perspective it might be seen as important because it is a means of maintaining a membership in a commercial centre. However, scientific research carried out to date holds no definite answers on the role of resistance training for fat loss, or indeed to indicate that it may be more relevant to use this than another less vigorous activity. Several studies show an increase in metabolic rate with resistance training in obese people, but other studies show no effect. Some show decreases in body fat levels while others do not. To date there has been little if any conclusive research comparing the two forms of activity over a set period of time in a homogeneous group of individuals.

## Forms of resistance training

There are many different paradigms for exercise, including resistance training, depending on the end goals (Table 13.5)

It has been supposed, as shown in Table 13.5, that the most effective type of resistance training for fat loss would be that requiring aerobic energy use, e.g. circuit training. Circuit training is the combination of a range of exercises carried out with light weights but with many repetitions to increase aerobic benefit. There seems to be little argument that this form of exercise would have fat burning benefits. Because it also involves muscular resistance, it could additionally provide metabolic benefits if in no

**Table 13.5: Exercise parameters for different goals**

| | Competitive sport | Cardio-vascular fitness | Fatness | Power | Muscle strength | Bulk | Flexibility |
|---|---|---|---|---|---|---|---|
| Frequency | 2–3 times daily | 3–4 days/week | 6–7 days/week | Varies in season | Alternate days | Alternate days | Regularly |
| Intensity | Up to maximum | 60–80% max. | 40–60% max. | 40–80% max. | Max. | 60–80% max. | Very low |
| Time | Very long total time : 3–5 hours | Relatively short: 30 mins | Long: 1+ hours | Short | Long | Long | Short–medium |
| Type | Sport related totally planned | Aerobic/anaerobic planned | Aerobic only (a) planned (b) incidental | Resistance | Resistance | Resistance | Stretching |
| Continuity | Intervals | Interval/continuous | Continuous | N/A | Intermittent | N/A | N/A |
| Speed | Generally fastest | Medium | Slow | Very fast | Slow–medium | Slow–medium | Very slow |

other way than in reducing the loss of muscle mass that may occur through diets alone.[15]

The main questions that remain about circuit training are the appropriate duration, intensity and frequency for optimal fat loss. Based on substrate utilisation, it would appear that the intensity should be moderate (i.e. around 40–60 per cent $VO_2$ max), and the duration as long as possible. Because many muscle groups are thought to require at least 48 hours to recover from the micro-cellular damage that results from resistance exercises, it would be inadvisable to carry out circuits, at least with high resistance, on a daily basis. Yet significant fat loss requires regular physical activity over long durations, so circuit training should be combined with other aerobic activities, such as walking, at least on every other day, but possibly also on circuit training days.[16]

It is more difficult to theorise about the effects of other types of resistance training. Resistance exercises for strength, body building or power all depend primarily on the phosphate and lactate energy systems. While there may be some aerobic involvement, and thus significant fat utilisation over an extended training session, it could be expected that this would be limited, particularly when compared with specific aerobic exercise. Hence, arguments for the use of this type of training for fat loss boil down to the expected changes in metabolic rate that might occur through maintenance or increase of muscle mass.

Metabolic changes due to muscle gain or maintenance might be expected to take two forms. In the first place, if there is a gain in muscle size in resistance-trained obese people, there is likely to be a gain in energy use due to this increase. Several studies have shown an increase in muscle size, or at least a maintenance of muscle mass due to resistance training in obese people, with or without energy restriction.[17] The increased effect on energy use, however, should not be expected to be great.

The second form may be more important, i.e. the reduction in decline of metabolism that would be expected to occur with loss of total body mass due to food restriction. This can amount to between 5–25 per cent within three weeks on a program using diet alone. If this decline is arrested by resistance training, as it has been shown to do with aerobic exercise, it could have a significant impact on total fat loss. However, to date the appropriate research has not been done in this area.

It is important to point out here that because we are talking about increasing, or at least maintaining muscle mass, this is likely to be reflected in weight *gain*, even though there may be some *fat* loss. Hence, use of the scales in this instance is definitely contra-indicated. For most obese people an increase in muscle density and weight, irrespective of fat loss, indicates an increase in body *size*, which is not generally desired by those looking for a decrease in overall body mass. The main question becomes whether it is more time efficient to carry out long, less vigorous, continuous aerobic exercise in the time that might otherwise be used for resistance training.

In the first place, many obese or overfat people by definition have, or are likely to have, reduced muscular efficiency. They are also likely to have decreased cardiovascular function. Hence, sudden intense activity such as resistance training may be both difficult and dangerous. It would not seem prudent, therefore, to put someone on a resistance training program at the outset of any fat loss regime.

Secondly, there is the issue of motivation. Many people have become fat because of their dislike of the traditional forms of exercise which underly weight training. While they may see themselves walking for fat loss, weight training may not be seen as a preferred option. Third, as mentioned above, there is the question of body perception. Finally, frequency of exercise is important. Because resistance training should not be carried out every day (unless a routine is 'split' i.e. upper body one day and lower body the next), it would be difficult to get the amount of exercise required (without becoming bored) if resistance training only was used for fat loss.

Having said this, it should be recognised that there may be some individuals, men in particular, who would prefer this type of activity instead of, or in addition to, aerobic activity. If so, they should be encouraged to combine both. Fitness centres can no longer expect to maintain their overfat clientele by programming a limited amount of exercise in the gym on alternate days. Consideration has to be given to the individual carrying out their own routines at times outside the gym setting and this should be supported and monitored by fitness centre personnel.

## IMPLICATIONS

1. A range of factors including gender, age, race, initial level of obesity, diet and genetic influences need to be considered in the prescription of specific physical activity programs for fat loss.
2. Patients with a genetic predisposition to obesity or with a long

history of obesity should have their previous exercise history carefully considered before any prescription as to the type of planned physical activity is given.

3. More attention needs to be given to duration, frequency and intensity of physical activity with pre-menopausal women and particularly those with gynoid-form obesity.

4. Greater attention needs to be paid to the combination of diet and physical activity in the case of long term obesity.

5. More emphasis should be placed on energy input in the initial stages of severe obesity with activity limited to incidental activity or weight-supportive exercise.

6. Consideration needs to be given to the different fat loss responses to exercise in post-menopausal compared to pre-menopausal women, and in android compared to gynoid forms of overfatness.

7. There is a need for greater attention to spontaneous activity in older patients. This tends to decline naturally and may do so even further after the introduction of a planned, daily physical activity session.

8. Different levels of intensity of physical activity may be required for clients with different levels of cardiovascular fitness.

9. It should not be assumed that individuals of equal fatness have equivalent cardiovascular fitness. Prescription needs to be specific to each individual.

10. For programs that are gym or fitness centre based, provision needs to be made for organised physical activity on days when the gym is not used (i.e. making up a total of 6–7 days/week of organised physical activity).

11. It should be recognised that total energy use and substrate utilisation can vary between individuals depending on gender and age. These variables need to be recognised in developing any individualised prescription.

12. It should be recognised that many people over-estimate the amount of physical activity they carry out during the course of a day. Hence, activity diaries, or pedometers or other measurement tools are suggested to keep track of daily efforts.

# VII
# MODERATORS

# 14

# Physiological adjustment and maintenance of fat loss

### SUMMARY OF MAIN POINTS

- Plateaus in fat loss are common and are due to physiological adjustments and reversion towards old habits.
- Maintenance of fat loss can be extremely difficult due to changes in metabolic rate and body composition.
- Physiological adjustments result in a lower than predicted loss of body fat with changes in energy balance.
- Adaptations include decreases in metabolic rate, changes in body composition, changes in fat utilisation and modifications of food intake.
- Long term maintenance of fat loss is highest amongst those who exercise regularly, change lifetime eating patterns and have well-developed stress management techniques.
- Plateaus may be countered by change.

As most perennial dieters will tell you, it's easy to lose fat, but keeping it off is another matter. If fat losses continued in direct proportion to the initial energy deficit (i.e. energy in minus energy out, as proposed in earlier models of fat loss), there would be a steady decline towards a goal (as shown in Figure 14.1), given a constant deficit in energy balance, but this is seldom the case. In reality, most fat loss occurs in the fashion of the upper line in Figure 14.1. There is an initial significant loss, then the rate of decline decreases until a type of 'plateauing' occurs followed often by a return to baseline levels. The challenge is to determine why this is so and if and how this can be modified.

Undoubtedly part of the reason for plateaus and regain is a return to previous habits. People tend to start fat loss programs with great gusto and commitment, but after 3 to 6 months their exercise and dietary habits tend to start slipping back. This is common and understandable given the environment of high-fat foods and labour-saving devices they face. To swim against this environmental tide takes effort and the effort is greater for those more genetically predisposed to obesity. It is not surprising that the effort fades with time. People often find it difficult to admit to a return to old habits and seek metabolic explanations for their plateaus. In truth, for most people the plateaus are due to a combination of behavioural and metabolic factors.

The extent to which metabolic changes slow down fat loss is a matter of some considerable debate. In 1950, the US nutritionist Dr Ancel Keys, wrote: 'It might seem entirely reasonable that the energetic processes of the body diminish in intensity as the exogenous food supply is reduced. It is reasonable in the sense that a wise man reduces his expenditure when his income is cut.'[1]

This survival tactic has been well-described in animal models of obesity. Studies at Cambridge University on a particular species of desert mouse for example, have shown that when compared with a 'city' mouse—or one accustomed to plenty of food—the desert mouse is able to adapt to decreases in body weight caused by lack of sustenance by simply slowing down its metabolic processes.[2] Humans have less facility to actively alter metabolic processes to match changes in food intake, although adaptations do certainly occur.

## PHYSIOLOGICAL ADAPTATIONS TO SLIMMING

The loss of body fat can lead to a range of physiological outcomes which, in turn, affect the further loss of body fat. Physiological adaptation to weight and fat loss can be divided into predictable changes (such as the decline in RMR in response to the loss of lean mass) and adaptive changes (where the body actively works to reduce the rate of weight loss). Dr Rudy Leibel and his colleagues from Rockefeller University in New York have tried to quantify the adaptive changes in lean and obese people as they lose weight.[3] For a 10 per cent weight loss, they found that total energy expenditure declined by about 450kcal, of which about

**Figure 14.1: Actual versus theoretical rates of fat loss over time**

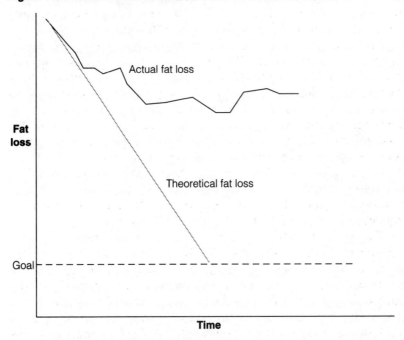

half could be explained by the changes in body composition and half could be considered adaptive. Table 14.1 summarises the results from this and other studies showing the elements which make the changes predictable and the level of evidence for adaptive changes beyond that.

## Physical responses

In a comprehensive review of the issue in 1991, Dr Andrew

**Table 14.1: Physical adaptations to slimming**

| Physical response | Reason | Added adaptation |
|---|---|---|
| ↓ Total energy expenditure (EE) | ↓ Fat-free mass (FFM) ↓ Weight | Yes (about 5%) |
| ↓ Resting metabolic rate (RMR) | ↓ Fat-free mass | Yes (about 50–150kcals) |
| ↓ Exercise | ↓ Weight | Yes (about 150–300kcals) |
| ↓ Thermic effect of food (TEF) | ↓ Calorie intake | No evidence |
| ↑ Appetite | Negative energy balance | Uncertain |
| ↓ Fat burning | ↓ Fat mass (FM) | Yes |

Prentice and his associates at the Dunn Clinical Nutrition Centre in Cambridge, identified the physiological outcomes of slimming.[4] These included: energy sparing adaptations, alterations in fat and lean body mass, altered energy substrate handling, changes in appetite, health related outcomes such as fitness and glucose tolerance, altered hormonal status, and altered fertility. These changes with slimming may also be moderated by a number of influences including genotype, degree of obesity at the onset of slimming, rate and duration of weight loss, composition of the slimming diet, use or non-use of exercise in the slimming regime and the influence of drugs if these are used.

Since many of the physiological adjustments are dependent on changes in body composition, we will first examine that before considering the adaptations themselves.

*Body composition*

Major changes in body composition occur with loss of body mass. Lean and fat tissue are almost inevitably lost together, although the proportions of each will differ widely. The greater the energy deficit and the lower the initial body fat level, the greater will be the percentage of fat-free mass (FFM) or muscle mass lost as the percentage of total weight loss.

Figure 14.2, adapted from Prentice, shows what happens. The vertical axis represents changes in the ratio of FFM to total body weight. A measure at the lower end of the scale suggests that FFM (muscle mass) to total weight loss is minimal. A measure of 0.2, for example, means that 20 per cent of the total weight loss is muscle. A measure of 0.8 on the other hand means 80 per cent of the weight lost is muscle and 20 per cent fat. The horizontal axis represents the starting level of body fatness.

The curves on Figure 14.2 show that people starting a diet with a low amount of body fat will lose most of their body mass in the form of muscle. Those starting with a high proportion of body fat on the other hand could be expected to only lose about 20 per cent in the form of muscle and the rest in the form of

---

MYTH-INFORMATION
*Individual foods such as grapefruit have been claimed to have special 'fat burning' potential. There is no physiological reason why this is so, nor any positive evidence to this effect.*

---

**Figure 14.2: Changes in fat-free mass (FFM) to total body weight (BW) loss after dieting**

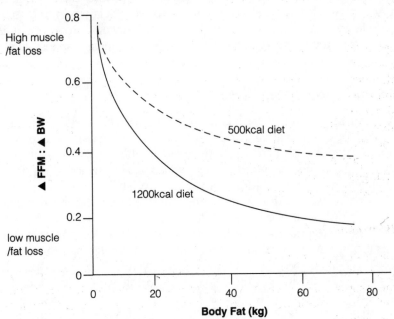

*Source:* Adapted from Prentice et al. (1991)[4]

fat. In other words, dieting for someone who is not carrying a lot of body fat is likely to result in significant losses of lean tissue. This illustrates the potential dangers in a lean or muscular person trying to lose extra fat by dieting alone, as is often the case with dieting women in particular.

For a very fat person, on the other hand, dieting is likely to be more effective for fat loss because of the greater stores available.

A more restrictive diet (500kcal v 1200kcal, Figure 14.2) will result in a greater proportion of lean mass being lost because the body simply cannot pull large amounts of energy out of the fat stores in a hurry. The lean mass represents the 'quick release' calorie compartment of the body so more energy is taken from the breakdown of muscle tissue. General estimates for ratios of lean to fat mass loss by obese people on reasonable diets according to English obesity expert Dr John Garrow, are about 25:75, i.e. 25 per cent lean body mass (LBM) to 75 per cent fat loss.[5] This is used as the standard estimate for big people.

*Counteracting body composition changes* Exercise is usually promoted as a means of reducing FFM losses to a minimum. Prentice and his colleagues cite eleven studies which were carried out to 1991, nine of which show exercise to be effective in reducing muscle loss. There have been many more since.[6,7] However, it is likely that the more restrictive the dietary regimen, the less likely FFM losses will be reduced by exercise.

*Energy/fat sparing adaptations*

As seen in Chapter 2, fat has a protective role for survival. Studies carried out with native African women show that they can lose up to 50 per cent of their body mass in the hungry season and then regain this in good times, without any major long term ill-effects. However, in doing so, the body shifts to a lower level of body mass including FFM and this reduces the resting and non-resting metabolic rates.

One extrapolation of the effects of adaptations is that the metabolism might become 'fixed' in its energy/fat sparing mode from repeated weight loss and gain cycles. This is popularly expressed as an increasing difficulty in losing weight and increasing ease of regaining weight with each cycle. Usually these series of *weight cycles* take place over a period of several decades and the effects of increasing age on weight loss and gain may well explain most of this phenomenon. There is no evidence that the metabolism gets permanently stuck in an energy/fat sparing mode, but then again getting evidence to prove or disprove the hypothesis is very difficult. The theory, however, has been popularised by Cannon and Einzig in their best selling book *Dieting Makes You Fat*,[8] and is also expressed in several recent 'anti-dieting' approaches. It is thus important to understand the extent of adaptation that occurs and possible ways of counteracting this.

Prentice and his group have studied energy sparing adaptations from a range of different energy level diets and concluded that the decrease in metabolic rate resulting from dieting, generally varies between 15–25 per cent. This is obviously large enough to slow down any ongoing fat loss. The decrease in metabolic rate is also generally proportionately greater than the decrease in body weight (at least in the early stages by about 3:1). The curve shown in Figure 14.3 shows the average decrease in metabolic rate resulting from dietary restrictions over time. Not unexpectedly, this curve is similar to reductions in body weight that occur with dietary restriction.

The changes in metabolic rate are probably mediated by a reduction in circulating thyroid hormone tri-iodothyrine (T3) and

**Figure 14.3: Decreases in resting metabolic rate (RMR) with weight loss**

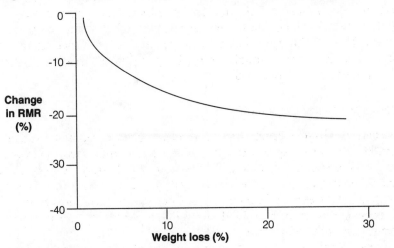

*Source:* Prentice et al. (1991)[4]

reductions in sympathetic nervous system activity. Thyroid hormone has been used to try to counteract the decline in RMR, but it has had so many negative effects on reducing muscle mass and causing medical problems that it is now not used for this purpose.

Prentice's group have carried out a theoretical analysis on the long term effects on body weight of a number of different energy level diets. The graphs in Figure 14.4 show the extent of weight loss both while on the diet, and while on a 1900kcal maintenance program. Although less weight is lost in the diet phase of this analysis on a 1000kcal diet, the total weight loss, after the maintenance period is not much less than from a 700kcal or 400kcal diet. The bottom line in the graph shows what might have happened on the very low 400kcal diet if, as many people miscalculate, no adaptation occurs.

It is presumed that adaptive responses will be more vigorous if the energy deficit is greater and weight loss is faster, although there is not a lot of evidence to back this up. The response, however, does seem to be proportionally greater in leaner people and this was observed by Ancel Keys (whose quote is at the beginning of this chapter) who studied the metabolic responses to semi-starvation in lean men who were staging a hunger strike in the 1940s. He noted, as did Leibel, that one of the most marked adaptations to a significant negative energy balance is lethargy and a reduction in physical activity including spontaneous activity.

Dieting can elicit energy sparing adaptations almost immedi-

**Figure 14.4: Anticipated weight loss on a variety of diets, with and without energy sparing adaptations**

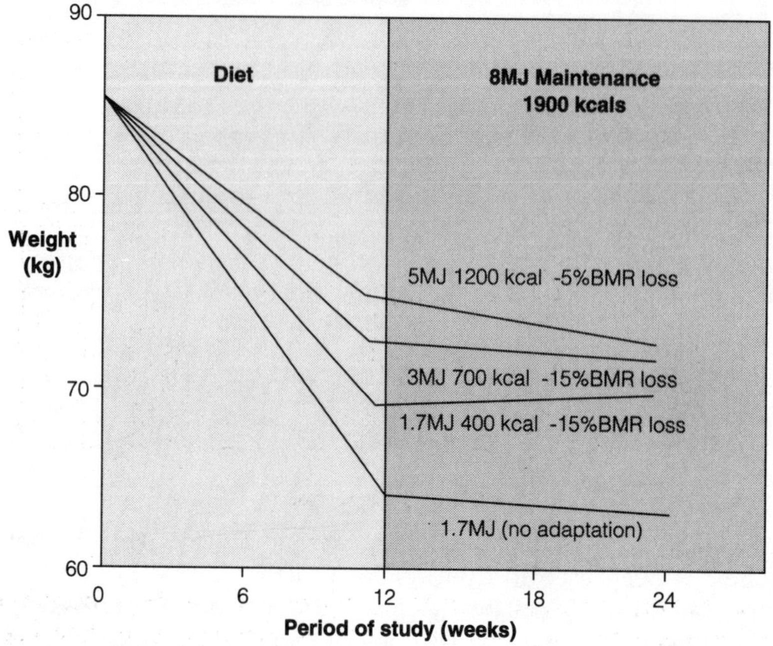

Source: Prentice et al. (1991)[4]

ately it is begun. Figure 14.5 shows the changes that occur over time to RMR during dieting and re-feeding (i.e. gradually increasing the food intake over time). There is an immediate decrease in RMR of around 5 per cent on day 1 of a diet. This continues at a decreasing rate over time to around 15–25 per cent. On re-feeding, as can be seen from the shaded bar on the right of figure 14.5, there is again an immediate jump in metabolic rate of around 5 per cent. This helps to explain the positive benefits

MYTH-INFORMATION

*Many weight control gimmicks capitalise on the technology of the day. Slow releasing 'fat burning' patches are a 1990s phenomenon following the apparent success of similar patches for smoking, diabetes etc. Unfortunately, the substance released (usually a seaweed extract) from diet patches has absolutely no proven effect on fat loss.*

**Figure 14.5: Changes in resting metabolic rate with dieting and re-feeding**

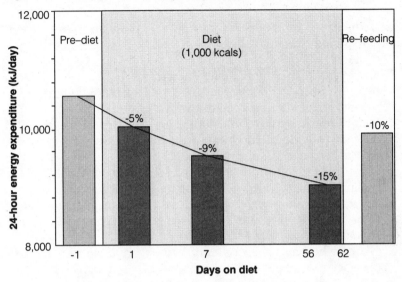

*Source:* Prentice et al. (1991)[4]

of re-feeding, particularly in cases where patients have been on very low calorie diets for long periods. Gradual re-feeding can actually help them to lose fat, at least up to a certain point (which is probably around 1200–1500kcal per day) due to this gradual reduction of energy sparing and its effects on metabolism.

*Counteracting energy sparing adaptations*

The main way of counteracting the adaptive reductions in energy expenditure is through physical activity. This has been shown in several studies to counteract the energy sparing effects of dietary restriction. It does this by increasing energy expenditure both during and after exercise and by maintaining lean body mass. Studies examining exercise, however, have not always been convincing, possibly due to the difficulty in getting people to comply with the exercise regimens that have been set for them. There is still enough evidence to suggest that exercise can help with those who do comply and indeed may be the most effective form of continuing fat loss in the maintenance stage. There is little argument amongst scientists that diet appears to have the *most immediate effect* on fat loss, but it is now also becoming increasingly clear that exercise should be the mainstay in *any fat loss maintenance program.*

217

## IMPLICATIONS

1. Maintenance requirements in a fat loss program may be more demanding and may differ significantly from actions leading to initial fat loss.

2. Energy restricting diets alone should not be used for fat loss over an extended period as these lead to physiological adaptations which can counteract the fat loss.

3. Energy restriction below 1200kcal per day should not be used over an extended period except in special cases of supervised dietary restriction for severe obesity.

4. Except where contra-indicated, physical activity should play a significant role in long term maintenance of fat loss.

5. Resistance training may be indicated in the maintenance stage of a fat loss program to ensure a counterbalance to the adaptations that occur to slimming.

6. Clients who have been on very low energy diets for extended periods may need to be gradually re-fed until daily energy intake is around 1200–1500kcal per day.

7. Clients should be made aware that long term continuous fat losses will only occur with increased changes in energy balance and/or alterations to the type of food intake and energy output.

8. The proportion of LBM to fat loss following a diet is likely to be much higher in people with a lower initial body fat level, hence people who are only mildly overfat and who use dietary restriction alone to treat this, are actually likely to finish with an higher proportion of body fat than at the start of a slimming initiative.

9. Physical activity should form a more significant part of the initial fat loss and fat loss maintenance regimes of those with a relatively low fat to total body mass ratio.

10. Behaviour modification principles utilised for fat loss should be continued in the maintenance stage.

# VIII
# INFLUENCES

# 15

# Environmental influences

SUMMARY OF MAIN POINTS

- Modern technological environments are associated with large increases in obesity in Western countries.
- Environments which influence overfatness can be categorised on size ('macro' or 'micro') and type ('physical' and 'socio-cultural').
- Macro environments represent the broader national and international perspective; micro environments are within the immediate family, friends and community.
- Environmental modifications are necessary for decreases in obesity at the population level and without these there are likely to be few major inroads made into the increasing prevalence of obesity.

The influence of the environment on obesity was eloquently shown in a study of six villages in Papua New Guinea.[1] Professor Paul Zimmett and his colleagues from Melbourne University developed an index of 'modernity' to measure how much modern technology was used in a particular population and to see if this is related to obesity levels. The 'modernity' index included measures of new technology use such as television and motor vehicles, education levels, occupation, father's employment, years living in an urban centre and type of housing. The Melbourne team then graded the six villages on their total 'modernity' scores and correlated these with obesity levels as measured by body mass index (BMI). As the level of 'modernity' increased in a village, so did the level of fatness of the population. They concluded that while modern technology is something we might all strive towards for improved quality of life, it has significant side effects on health. This is due particularly to the decreases in physical activity, as well as the increased availability of high energy dense foods, particularly fatty processed foods.

The current environment in modern society in relation to obesity can be compared with that associated with cigarette smoking in the 1960s and 1970s. While individual and group 'quit' smoking programs had reasonable success at the individual level, they had little impact on smoking rates in most Western countries until population-wide measures were taken and public attitudes towards smoking changed. Legislation on smoke-free environments, advertising bans, price hikes and a range of other environmental changes have all been major contributors to the decreases in smoking.[2]

There are a number of different environments—macro, micro, physical and socio-cultural—in which human beings operate. These, in turn, can affect aspects of fat/energy input (F/EI) such as food supply or availability, or fat/energy expenditure (F/EE), such as facilities for, and attitudes to, physical activity. A summary of some of the main influences is given in Table 15.1.

## THE MACRO ENVIRONMENT

The macro environment refers to the wider physical and social aggregate of conditions or influences on an individual. At the upper level, this represents the world, and the influences of modern communication systems and technology. At the lower level it refers to national or cultural based influences over which the individual has little or no control. As mentioned above, within both the macro and micro environments there are physical and socio-cultural influences.

### The physical macro environment

Influences on body fatness in the wider physical environment include the food supply, availability of facilities for physical activity, and the demands for physical activity for day-to-day living. The food supply within a population is influenced by a number of

**Table 15.1: Some examples of environmental influences on obesity**

| Size of environment | Type of environment | | | |
| --- | --- | --- | --- | --- |
| | Physical | | Socio-cultural | |
| | EI (Food) | EE (Exercise) | EI (Food) | EE (Exercise) |
| Macro | • Food supply<br>• Storage<br>• Availability<br>• Food outlets<br>• Economy<br>• Advertising<br>• Legislation<br>• Pricing<br>• Taxation | • Technology<br>• Transport<br>• Facilities<br>• Urbanisation<br>• School PE<br>• Weather<br>• Street lighting<br>• Street safety | • Advertising<br>• Attitudes<br>• Fast food<br>• Business lunch<br>• Festivities<br>• Male attitudes<br>• Customs<br>• Food fashions | • Social trends<br>• Recreation time<br>• Attitudes to physical activity<br>• Recreation fashions |
| Micro | • Food at home<br>• Accessibility<br>• Meal sizes<br>• Low-fat foods<br>• Leftovers<br>• Budget<br>• Cooking skills | • Second cars<br>• Remote TVs<br>• Electronics<br>• Exercise equipment | • Gender influence<br>• Weekly habits<br>• Social circles<br>• Family patterns<br>• Work and peer influences | • Attitudes and support of:<br>  peers<br>  family<br>  partners<br>• Reducing inactivity in kids |

factors including agricultural practices, pricing and taxation structures, manufacturing and food processing, marketing and the availability of distribution outlets as well as the general economy. Supply is ultimately affected, however, by Government policy and public demand.

Meat and livestock producers were traditionally rewarded for fatter carcasses by having prices determined by total weight and/or fat content. Dairy producers also received greater incomes from higher milk fat content. However, public demand for lower-fat products has caused a shift away from prices based on fat. The public shift towards chicken meant an increase in the production of poultry. This led to an increase in battery hen farming, and as a result of the reduced activity of the birds (which were previously free range), the fat content of poultry seems to have increased significantly.

In the meantime, public demand led other meat producers to significantly reduce the fat content of their product, through different farming, butchering and marketing practices. Lean pork, beef and lamb are now highly comparable with poultry in fat content, and in some cases, lower in fat. Hence changes in the food supply can influence changes in the availability and use of products likely to facilitate increases in obesity and this has become a targeted activity of the public health lobby.[3]

MYTH-INFORMATION

*Eye-glasses that make food look unappetising
are one of a number of weird products
designed to attract the weight control dollar.
Unfortunately, eating behaviour is stimulated
by a little more than just vision.*

Food processing and supply is also influenced by the market place and public policy. Requirements for labelling of fat content of packaged foods accompanied by public education campaigns aimed at increasing awareness of fattening and non-fattening products, can help reduce their demand and in turn put pressure on food producers to modify the supply. Programs like 'Pick the Tick'[4] also bring nutrition into the equation for manufacturers and making the product eligible to achieve the tick endorsement becomes the goal for which manufacturers can aim.

Fast food outlets have increased their turnover dramatically in Western countries, with an estimated 1 in 3 meals now reportedly purchased outside the home. Per capita consumption of takeaway foods has increased by 10 per cent per year since 1984, with a total annual market in Australia in 1994 of $5 billion. Approximately $540 per capita is also spent per year on snack foods, compared to $506 on fruit and vegetables.[5] Government policy in the form of incentives, as well as disincentives (such as taxes) for the production and sale of reduced-fat takeaways is one future option to slow down the increases in obesity.

Public education campaigns are also necessary at this level to help develop skills for choosing and preparing food. A very important accompaniment to such education efforts are attempts to improve the food choice in places where people eat, such as school and work canteens, lunch bars and institutions such as hospitals and boarding schools. Even small changes, such as not automatically buttering baked goods, may have a major impact, simply because of the volume of people eating in these settings, and work to this effect must be a priority for health authorities.

The options for energy/fat expenditure in a society can also be influenced at a macro environmental level. As technology advances, with increases in the number and type of effort saving devices both in the workplace and in the community, the need for daily movement is reduced. The development of motor vehicles and other transport options, for example, has reduced the need to walk. For many people, men in particular, the work environment offered the main opportunity for physical activity. Even twenty to thirty years ago many jobs required some degree of physical effort, but the development and increasing sophistication of machinery continues to reduce this significantly. Decrease in work place activity is often given as one of the main reasons for the increases in fatness of working class men in recent times. It's interesting to note that only a little more than twenty years ago, white collar workers were generally fatter than blue collar workers. But in some 'blue collar' areas like industrial cities, 3 in 4 men are now regarded as overweight or obese compared to 1 in 4 amongst 'white collar' men.[6]

Some form of physical activity has been a requirement for survival and day-to-day living for most of human history. Famous Swedish exercise physiologist Per-Olaf Aastrand has pointed out that if the whole of human history over 460 million years was regarded as a race of 460 kilometres, only the last 10mm would have been covered by a 100-year-old man living today.[7] The period during which machinery has taken away the need for physical effort has really only been the last 40–50 years, or 2–3mm on the 460km journey of the human race!

As the need for physical activity in day-to-day life has decreased, such activity has become increasingly institutionalised through the development of the modern fitness industry, however, the use of a gym for 30 minutes a couple of times a week probably doesn't compensate for the decrease in spontaneous physical activity during the rest of the week. The idea of a fitness centre also has limited appeal to many people, particularly those who are excessively fat, and figures show that only 1–2 per cent of the population actually use these facilities on a regular basis.

In schools, the presence or absence of physical education (PE) classes and facilities for physical activity through play can influence the early development of obesity. Where physical education was once compulsory in Australia, this is now often left to the discretion of individual schools. Trials with a compulsory daily PE program in South Australian primary schools in the 1980s showed that this not only decreased body fat and improved measures of health in young children but also aided academic performance.[8] The growth in childhood obesity is now leading to a re-evaluation of the need for PE by education authorities in some parts of the world.

Finally, the increasing urbanisation of the population has, in many cases, led to a decreased opportunity for increased energy expenditure. Where there are facilities such as walking paths, bike tracks, or other recreational facilities, but no street lighting, there are often concerns about personal safety, particularly for women and children. Positive changes to the macro environment to increase daily energy expenditure will need to include provision at the national and local Government level for safe recreational facilities. Indeed, possibly the best way to motivate individuals to increase activity is to present them with easy exercise choices.

If the fitness industry is to participate in fat loss there will also need to be a significant change in its image. New facilities are currently being developed in some countries that de-emphasise the fitness and 'body beautiful' aspects of exercise that are de-motivational for so many people, but allow opportunities for safe, regular, low intensity, long duration activities such as treadmill walking, cycling and stair climbing, accompanied by electronic entertainment such as videos, TVs, and stereos.

## The socio-cultural macro environment

The socio-cultural macro environment represents the values, expectations and attitudes of the wider social environment. Community attitudes to convenience foods and leisure saving technologies are examples. A hedonistic and materialistic atmosphere where moderation is considered unfashionable is common in many sectors of Western societies. Where this is coupled with easy access to palatable, high-fat foods and reduced necessity for energy expenditure, obesity levels are likely to increase. In Australia, an advertising expenditure of $1million per day on food stuffs, confectionery and soft drinks is combatted by an equivalent amount *per year* spent on public health education, some of which is presumably aimed at eating for reduced body fatness.

With increased affluence there is also an increased opportunity for over-indulgence through the social processes of dining out, business lunches, social festivities and celebrations. There are also cultural and ethnic differences in food preferences and exercise availability: European-style food is usually higher in fat, for example, than Asian foods; some foods, such as pork, have traditionally held a higher social status than vegetables or fruit in different cultures; opportunities for exercise are reduced for some ethnic and religious groups such as Middle Eastern and Muslim women.

Male attitudes to health are known to differ from those of females. Men have typically been less responsive to health messages, attend doctors less often, but suffer more from most forms of illness than women. This has been attributed to social and attitudinal differences between the sexes—men feel more isolated and vulnerable if they admit any concern about their health.[9] Overcoming these attitudes is a major obstacle to providing acceptable fat loss programs for men. Cultural attitudes in some ethnic groups also mean that partner support for fat loss practices, particularly by males for females, is low or non-existent.

Social attitudes to physical activity can influence participation. Increased interest in jogging in the 1970s for example, followed by aerobics and then weight training in the 1980s, formed the pattern of a social 'trend'. It is doubtful, however, if these have compensated for the decreases in physical activity that have occurred at the workplace or the decreases in other 'incidental' activity in day-to-day life. Multi-event sports like triathlons have become popular, but this is usually only amongst the very fit. Fun runs and community activities, however, have the potential to attract large numbers of people who may otherwise remain inactive. Socially acceptable forms of activity differ according to ethnic group, nationality, age and gender. Being fat carries a negative status, but more so for women, and being inactive also carries a negative status, but more so for men.

### MYTH-INFORMATION

*One brand of slim fit shorts advertises that the product '. . . uses heat and micro massage to promote the removal of waste and draws super-fluous fat and water molecules from the skin's surface'. If true, this would require the product to be registered under the Pharmaceutical Services Act.*

The influence of the socio-cultural macro environment has been particularly noticeable in countries like the UK and the Netherlands. The overall nutrient intake in the food in both countries is similar, but the obesity rate in Britain is increasing at a much greater rate than in Holland. According to Dr Wim Saris, from the University of Limburg, this might be put down simply to the fact that only 3 per cent of British transport involves the bicycle, whereas the equivalent figure is over 30 per cent in the Netherlands.[10]

### THE MICRO ENVIRONMENT

The micro environment refers to those aspects of the environment that are closer to the individual. Again, these can be classed as either physical or socio-cultural. Because they are more personal, however, they are much more amenable to change and represent opportunities for those working at the clinical or individual level. Many potential micro-environmental changes, either within the home, workplace or social environment, are often considered within a behaviour therapy approach to obesity management.

### The physical micro environment

Most changes at the macro-environmental level require wide changes such as in government policy, food industry practices or the promotion of healthy choice by food marketers. However, at the individual level it is possible to 'psychologically immunise' individuals against the counter-productive influences of the environment through education, counselling and behaviour change practices. The idea of avoiding fast foods, reducing the availability or accessibility of fatty foods in the home and walking instead of using automated transport, all help to reduce the negative effects of the macro environment or micro environment, although it must be emphasised that these have to be continually reinforced to maintain effectiveness.

Foods coming into the home can be limited through the teaching of appropriate shopping skills—reading labels, purchase of alternative low-fat products and providing tips for shopping such as never shopping on an empty stomach. Members of the family can be encouraged to participate in local sporting activities, to walk to the shop for the paper rather than taking the car or to join in a family bike ride or bush walk. The overuse of energy-saving devices can be easily controlled within the home. All these efforts can help to maintain a healthier micro environment. A home audit such as that shown in Table 15.2 can be a useful guide to micro-environmental changes for body fat reductions.

In many cases the environment outside the home such as the work canteen or lunch bar can be influenced by one or two individuals and are therefore considered 'micro', rather than 'macro'. The impact of a 'School Canteen Project' is an example of a few influential people modifying the environment which in turn affects large numbers of school children.

### The socio-cultural micro environment

Partner support has been shown to be particularly important to

**Table 15.2: Example of a home audit for fat loss**

*A home 'audit' for fat loss*

Check the household for:
- high-fat foods (i.e. >10% fat) stored in the house
- accessibility of fatty snack foods and other 'treats'
- oversized meals presented at meal times
- availability of low-fat alternative products e.g. milk, cheese
- limited fats or oils for use in cooking
- low-fat cooking methods and machines available (e.g. microwave, grillers)
- easy access to fresh fruit
- excessive use of effort saving devices (e.g. remote control TV, electric toothbrushes, leaf blowers, electronic kitchenware, etc.)
- availability of bikes or exercise equipment
- limited eating places within the house

the success of fat loss programs in the home environment. It's often presupposed that family nutrition practices are influenced mostly by the female in the household, although one study done with spouses of men in a male 'waist loss' program in Australia has shown that there is a greater influence on the household environment when the man of the house decides to make a change to reduce fatness. It also seems that females are more likely to provide support for their male partner to lose fat than vice versa.[11]

There are regular eating and exercise patterns within families, workplaces and other social settings which may have counter-productive effects on fat loss programs. A recent survey of eating patterns, for example, showed that dietary patterns close to that regarded as healthy (such as eating breakfast and eating low-fat and high-fibre foods with limited alcohol consumption) are most common on Monday mornings. After that, the dietary pattern declines to Sunday nights with the worst consumption patterns occurring from Friday to Sunday.[12] Work and social pressures over the course of the week no doubt help cause this effect, which also occurs in a yearly cycle from early in the New Year until the end of the year. The implications of this are that fat loss programs designed to lead to lifestyle changes are less likely to be effective if introduced at those times (i.e. late in the week or year) when the social environment is least supportive.

With children, the influence of the family is most significant. Recent research by Dr Len Epstein, a psychologist working in childhood obesity in the US, has shown that reducing inactivity by rewarding children for *not* watching TV or carrying out other sedentary activities such as video games is a more effective fat loss technique than directly rewarding their involvement in exercise or sport. More importantly, many children who are encouraged to reduce inactivity actually end up liking exercise, and even vigorous exercise, more than those who are put into a regimented exercise program.[13]

Peer and close support group attitudes are also a significant part of the socio-cultural micro environment. For men in particular, it's thought that only exercise that is vigorous and exhaustive has value for improving health and reducing body fatness.[14] Exercise such as that required to walk to the shop, walk up stairs, mow the lawn, or carry out chores is seen purely as a nuisance, or inconvenience. A major initiative here is to change the mental orientation to regarding all forms of activity as an 'opportunity' rather than an 'inconvenience'. By reframing the issue in the minds of the subject, the significance of the external environment is, at least, partly nullified. Currently, this is not aided by social attitudes which regard someone as being successful once they possess all the leisure saving devices possible: while these remain a sign of economic affluence, they are undoubtedly facilitators of physical inactivity.

## PUBLIC HEALTH APPROACHES TO OBESITY

Prevention of obesity will only come about through major public health initiatives. By definition, these affect large parts of the population. The changes made, for example, in food labelling or workplace canteen policies complement and support public education programs. Changes in the macro environment and perhaps the physical micro environment are the most accessible for public health programs. Since it is changes in the macro environment which are the driving force behind the increasing obesity, we need to turn to the macro environment to look for solutions to the epidemic.

## IMPLICATIONS

1. There is a need to take a wider view of the causes of overfatness and obesity than simple fat and/or energy imbalances.
2. Examine the influences in both the macro and micro environment that limit an individual's ability to successfully reduce body fat; list these and attempt to plan counter approaches to them.

3. If possible, get spouses and partners involved in the modification of the micro environment for reducing body fat levels.
4. Keep fatty foods either out of the household environment, or not easily accessible.
5. Encourage the use of 'person power' through physical activity and 'incidental activity', rather than using machinery.
6. Modify the food supply at the micro-environmental level if this can't be changed at the macro level, e.g. through reading food labels, learning appropriate shopping techniques, etc.
7. Increase awareness of, and access to, facilities for increasing levels of physical activity such as recreation centres, parks, playgrounds, walkways, cycle tracks and stairways in buildings.
8. Encourage walking rather than the use of vehicles where possible (i.e. park away from the destination, walk up the stairs instead of using escalators).
9. Get group support to facilitate physical activity (e.g. walking with a friend or group).
10. Encourage an attitude which regards movement as an 'opportunity', rather than an 'inconvenience'.
11. Discourage the use of labour saving electronic equipment in the home such as remote controls for the TV, automatic garage doors, electronic can openers, toothbrushes etc.
12. Don't commence a fat loss program at times when social support is likely to be least, i.e. at the end of the week or end of the year in particular.
13. Recognise the potential for environmental change and support individual and public health programs.

# 16
# Biological influences

## SUMMARY OF MAIN POINTS

- Biological influences on obesity include age, sex, race, hormonal factors (such as puberty, pregnancy and menopause) and a wide range of genetic factors and interactions between these.
- Recent findings have isolated a number of genes associated with various aspects of obesity such as hunger and food preference.
- The propensity to store body fat increases with age, and there are important age by sex, and possibly racial interactions

As touched on in Chapter 7, there are multiple biological regulators of body fat. These are, in particular, genetics (including sex and race) and age. The extent to which these affect fatness levels and the implications for modifying programs are discussed below.

## GENETICS

The controversy about the influences of nature versus nurture has been going on for centuries. The last 20 years of the 20th century have seen tremendous advances in molecular sciences, which have enabled a greater appreciation of the importance of genetics in many areas of human biology. The human-genome project, which commenced in the 1980s, plans to map all human genes (a directory that will provide genetic 'addresses' equivalent to about eight major city phone books) by the year 2010. In the end, it is likely that what will be proven is what we have always known, that parents are responsible for a lot, including the degree of body fatness in their children. On the other hand, genetic influences do not necessarily imply pre-determination. The influence of a *genotype* (the genetic 'blueprint') which favours obesity will only be translated into the *phenotype* (the manifest characteristics of the genotype of an obese person) under certain conditions. Unlike having blue eyes or fair hair, the genetic expression of fatness is only manifest given the right conditions. In other words, an environment which favours energy surplus is virtually a prerequisite for the obesity genes to show themselves.

The studies of genotype and body fat are usually based on comparisons of body size in families and some of the most informative studies involve twins. Identical twins share 100 per cent of their genes, whereas non identical twins only share 50 per cent of their genes. By comparing the similarities in body size between the two types of twins, an estimate of the genetic contribution can be made. Three major twin studies carried out in the late 1980s showed some startling findings, in particular, amazing similarities in body fatness and body shape in identical twins who had been reared apart since birth, some never even having met! In general, genes explain about 25–40 per cent of the variation in body fatness, although it has to be remembered that these estimates are based on people living in fairly similar environments.

---

### MYTH-INFORMATION

*Because there are known genetic factors involved in body fatness, this does not imply that genetically prone individuals have to become fat. Genes for fatness are only manifest in the appropriate environment.*

---

Some of the most significant research in this area has come from Professor Claude Bouchard and his group at Laval University in Quebec.[1] Their experiments are carried out with pairs of twins who are kept in comfortable holiday-type accommodation for months at a time, and compare responses to various eating and exercise regimes. Their findings confirm that there is a wide range of responses to identical environmental influences and that the degree of response (such as the degree of weight gained for a given calorie excess) is largely genetically determined.

Genetic influences are unlikely to be the result of a single 'fat gene'. Genes probably influence all aspects of energy balance including food preferences, nutrient digestion and processing, fat burning and storage and physical activity levels. In fact, to the mid-1990s, a total of 24 genes had been specifically identified as related to some aspect of obesity, but scientists believe several hundreds more are likely to be involved.

One key factor which appears to be at least partly inherited, for example, is food preference. Researchers at the University of Cincinnati examined preferences for 17 different types of foods ranging from fruit to snacks, chips and hamburgers.[2] Comparisons were made between young (9–18-year-old) identical and non-identical twins living together. Frequency of eating and preferences for different foods were rated on a series of scales which indicated that genetic factors (e.g. in identical twins) do, indeed, appear to account for certain food preferences. The main heritable factor in preference appears to be sensitivity to, and preference for, bitter compounds in foods. Preferences for orange juice, broccoli, cottage cheese, chicken, sweetened cereal and hamburgers, for example, all appear to have an hereditary component.

## The satiety gene

All of the above suggests that obesity is a 'polygenic' disorder, or that there are a number of genetic components to obesity. Major excitement was aroused in scientific circles in late 1994 because of the identification of a gene apparently linked to 'switching' on and off hunger, called a satiety gene. The history of this discovery is fascinating and helps provide an understanding of the complexity of the problem.

It has been known for some time that substances must exist in the blood which signal the state of energy stores to the brain so that hunger can be turned on and off. In the early 1950s, a mechanism called an 'appestat' was hypothesised to operate like a thermostat in 'switching off' hunger after a certain level of food intake. This was further supported in the 1960s and 1970s by some ingenious research carried out by Dr Douglas Coleman at the Jackson Laboratory in Maine with two inbred strains of obese mice (called 'db' for diabetes and 'ob' for obese).[3] Coleman joined these mice with normal lean mice (a process called 'parabiosis')

## Figure 16.1: 'Parabiotic' mice and obesity

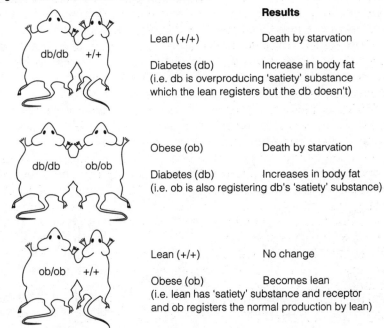

**Results**

Lean (+/+)        Death by starvation

Diabetes (db)        Increase in body fat
(i.e. db is overproducing 'satiety' substance
which the lean registers but the db doesn't)

Obese (ob)        Death by starvation

Diabetes (db)        Increases in body fat
(i.e. ob is also registering db's 'satiety' substance)

Lean (+/+)        No change

Obese (ob)        Becomes lean
(i.e. lean has 'satiety' substance and receptor
and ob registers the normal production by lean)

so they both had the same circulatory system (see Figure 16.1). In doing so, strange things happened.

When a normal mouse was joined with a 'db' strain mouse, the lean mouse actually starved to death—even in the presence of abundant food. This suggested that the 'db' strain had an over-supply of some substance in the blood to tell it to stop eating, but that this wasn't working in the 'db' mouse. When an 'ob' and a 'db' mouse were joined, the 'ob' mouse died from starvation, but the 'db' mouse increased its weight by over-eating. Again, this suggests that the 'db' mouse was over-supplying a 'switch off' substance which was not working with it, but which worked excessively well with the 'ob' mouse. Finally, when a normal mouse was joined with an 'ob' mouse, the 'ob' mouse lost weight and became normal. All this suggested that normal mice have a normal amount of a substance which the 'ob' mouse does not have, and which the 'db' mouse has too much of, but which has no effect (i.e. does not reach a receptor) in the 'db' mouse.

Dr Jeremy Friedman and his team from Rockefeller University in New York then isolated a gene which codes for the production of a protein from fat cells, which tells the brain when satiation has been reached.[4] The protein has since been identified, synthesised and injected into obese mice and found to reduce their body weight. The substance has been called 'leptin' (after the Greek word 'leptos' meaning 'thin'), and the race is now on to develop drugs which may be useful in human obesity.[5] Most scientists, however, warn that the discovery is not likely to be as simple a remedy as some have claimed, and that much more work still needs to be done.

There are likely to be few, if any, human equivalents of the ob or db mice which have major single gene abnormalities. In humans, there may however, be gene variations which result in some people being less able than others to switch off their appetite. Genetic influences in human obesity are indicated by some simple factors such as:

- Presence of lifetime or long term obesity in one or both parents. Studies have shown that the chances of being obese are around 80 per cent if both parents are obese, 40 per cent if one parent is obese and only 7 per cent if neither parent is obese.
- Presence of obesity since childhood. Genetically influenced obesity is usually manifest early in life, particularly before or around adolescence. For this reason someone who has always had a problem, particularly if the problem is also in the immediate family, is more likely to be genetically influenced.
- Presence of type I obesity. Abdominal obesity, particularly in men, is generally regarded as being environmentally determined. Ovoid-shaped fatness, together with the factors mentioned above, may suggest genotypical influences.

Although the factors mentioned above provide no certainty about genetic influence, they may give some indications that fat loss is likely to be a more difficult proposition in an individual who is genetically predisposed to fatness and that efforts to prevent fat gain may need to be lifelong; therefore, this person needs long term goals which are realistic. Special attention may also need to be given to hunger and behavioural cues and to maintenance of body weight after slimming (see Chapter 18). The questionnaire shown in Table 16.1 provides some indication of the heritability of fatness.

## SEX

There are major sex differences in body fat loss and maintenance ability. Some of the relevant differences between the sexes are listed in Table 16.2.

**Table 16.1: Genetic influences questionnaire**

| | | Score |
|---|---|---|
| 1. | As far as you know, were either or both of your parents significantly overweight for most of their lives? | |
| | Neither/don't know | 0 |
| | Yes, one parent | 1 |
| | Yes, both parents | 2 |
| 2. | Do you have any brothers or sisters who have been significantly overweight for most of their lives? | |
| | No | 0 |
| | Yes, one | 1 |
| | Yes, more than one | 2 |
| 3. | When did you first become overweight? | |
| | After 20 | 0 |
| | During my teens | 1 |
| | Before my teens | 2 |
| 4. | How difficult do you find it to take off weight? | |
| | Not difficult at all | 0 |
| | Reasonably difficult | 1 |
| | Very difficult | 2 |
| 5. | Where do you mainly get fat when you put on weight? | |
| | On the stomach | 0 |
| | On the hips and buttocks | 1 |
| | All over | 2 |

*Scores:* **0–4**: No apparent genetic involvement.
**5–7**: Moderate hereditary component.
**8–10**: There appears to be a significant hereditary component to your weight problem. This means you may need special help for effective weight loss.

As we have seen, male and female fat distribution and fat cell reactivity differs. Male-type centrally stored fat cells (around the abdomen) are known to be different in size and function to gluteal tissue, being more responsive to lipolytic and less responsive to lipogenic stimuli. Males generally use more energy for a set amount of exercise because of the larger proportion of lean body mass, or muscle, for a given body mass. Gluteal fat stores in females are widely regarded as having a biological function as an energy reserve for reproduction and milk production during lactation, and these are relatively resistant to fat loss even with high energy output or low energy intake.[6]

Women experience greater hormonal swings throughout life (menarche, menstrual cycle, pregnancy and menopause) and these can impact significantly on body fat levels. The hormone levels in men by contrast, change only gradually with time as testosterone levels gradually decline with age. Women who don't gain excessive weight during pregnancy, and who remain active both during pregnancy and after parturition, don't seem to be at risk for extra fat gain—at least for the first 1–2 pregnancies. Women who are overfat or obese and who gain excessive weight during pregnancy are more likely to have problems after delivery. Breast-feeding

**Table 16.2: Sex differences in fat loss factors**

| Males | Females |
|---|---|
| • Fat stored on the waist | • Fat stored on hips/buttocks |
| • Fat cells smaller | • Fat cells larger |
| • High rate of lipolysis | • High rate of lipogenesis |
| • More energy for exercise | • Less energy for exercise |
| • Lipolysis greater after fasting | • Fat more resistant to fasting |
| • Fat unaffected by reproduction | • Fat levels can change after pregnancies/menopause |
| • High metabolic rate | • Lower metabolic rate |
| • Heavy body image ideal | • Light body image ideal |

mothers (over 6 months of breast-feeding) have been shown to stay leaner for longer than non-breast feeding mothers. In general also, the more babies a woman has, the greater her chances of becoming overfat or obese. It's not known, however, whether this is due to physiological factors or the reduced ability to exercise and increased opportunity for over-eating, or whether it's simply an association with other socioeconomic factors. Large families and obesity are more common in lower socioeconomic groups and the social status may be the determining factor for both.[7]

> ### MYTH-INFORMATION
> *The notion that everyone responds in a similar fashion to the same diet program is now regarded as quite wrong. Biological, physiological and behavioural differences ensure that even in a similar environment, people are different!*

Body composition differences between the genders also favour males in terms of energy expenditure. Men, in general, have a higher lean body mass to total mass ratio, with 12–24 per cent of body composition in the form of adipose tissue. Females on the other hand carry 15–30 per cent of their body mass in the form of fat. Higher lean body mass, even given constant weight, ensures a higher resting metabolic rate and hence men tend to have a greater energy use at rest. During exercise it has been shown that a man utilises up to 40 per cent more energy walking a set distance than a similar sized female.[8]

Finally, there are psychological and sociological differences between the sexes which, although potentially changeable, can have a profound impact on body fat levels. The idealised female shape, for example, is now one of thinness. This has changed

throughout history, there being good evidence (in art and literature) that a more ample female form has been preferred in the
past. When fatness indicated wealth, a well-fed female body was
desired. In the 20th century in Western countries, where energy-
rich food is generally plentiful, fatness is easy and leanness is
more associated with wealth, status and influence. Anorexia
nervosa is the pathological extreme of this obsession with a thin
figure.

Dietitian Jenny O'Dea from Sydney University has shown that
females generally idealise a much thinner body size for themselves
than is preferred by most males. The social pressures to conform
to an ideal shape is greater in females (even if it is largely females
who apply that pressure). A pot belly in a male doesn't attract
the same social pressures as a similar degree of fatness in a female,
even though the male's fatness is more dangerous to health.

In contrast to the ideal female body form of thinness, the ideal
male body is generally bulkier, albeit bulk from muscles rather
than fat. The extreme version of this is seen in obsessive body
building and the eating disorders associated with this such as
excessively high protein diets and supplements. As an eating
disorder, this type of extreme has similarities to anorexia in females
with its obsession with body shape, distortion of body image and
extreme eating patterns.[9]

Sex differences in body fatness have very real implications for
fat loss planning. It is totally unrealistic to expect similar results
from a male and female placed on the same type of fat loss
program, although this is often expected by partners who may
undertake the same kind of program. To the extreme frustration
(and often guilt and depression) of the female partner, it is usually
the male who is able to lose fat more easily and faster, and to
keep this off longer, than the female. More support is often needed
for females to ensure adequate eating patterns to encourage
satisfaction with a body shape which is less than ideal and to
prevent discouragement with slow fat losses.

## RACE

Among the genetic factors thought to influence fat loss response,
racial differences have probably been studied least. Yet simple
observation shows that there are big differences in body shape
between Negroids, Asians and Caucasians in particular. Negroid
women store fat more readily around the hips and buttocks:
amongst Negroids, the Hottentot women of South Africa, who

have survived in a severe desert climate for millennia, are well-known for their exaggerated gynoid fat stores, which may have increased the survival potential of the race in the desert.

Asian women are known for their small hips. Waist-to-hip ratios used as a measure of risk in Caucasians, therefore, are generally not relevant for these women because they give measures more characteristic of a man. Other fat measures such as skinfolds or machine measures may be more relevant here, and particularly when comparing between racial groups. Normative values for body fat, therefore, need to take account of racial differences, but to date this has not been done.

The deposition of fat may also differ amongst racial groups. Chinese and Indians, for example, appear to put additional fat on the waist first before then filling out all over. Island races like Samoans and Tongans are big people and are prone to developing significant obesity, but that fat is stored more evenly over the body. Aboriginal Australians have naturally lean limbs and small hips but also a high tendency for fat gain from eating 'Western-style' foods. This appears to manifest more in the form of abdominal obesity rather than the overall obesity more common of Polynesians and Melanesians.


## AGE

New research on the effects of ageing on body fat suggest that there are a number of components of ageing which mean that gaining fat stores with age is a 'natural' process and that losing fat becomes more difficult. Changes with age that promote fat gain are:

- *a decrease in lean body mass:* and therefore a reduction in metabolic rate. This may be compensated for by such activities as resistance training, although the extent to which this can occur is not clear at this stage.[10] Metabolic rate is thought to decrease naturally by about 2 per cent per decade after the age of 20.
- *changes in fat oxidation:* The rate at which the body burns fat as an energy source in contrast to blood sugars, decreases with age, possibly as a result of the increase in body fat mass. This means fat is stored more readily and used less easily as a fuel source in the elderly.
- *changes in the influences of stimuli which 'break down' fat (lipolytic stimuli):* Hormones such as growth hormone and

240

testosterone all decrease with age and catecholamines from the adrenal glands appear less effective with age. Hence, the normal status of older people promotes fat gain.

- *decreases in spontaneous physical activity (SPA):* As well as a decrease in physical activity (through sport and games) it now appears that even if older people consciously exercise vigorously to lose fat, they may unconsciously decrease their rate of physical activity at other times during the day: they simply get more tired than young people as a result of exercise, and unless an effort is made to maintain SPA, the net effect may be no real gain in overall physical activity.
- *increased associated health conditions:* heart disease, arthritis and other muscular-skeletal problems.
- *a decrease in intra-muscular fat as an energy source:* There are significant stores of fat in muscle tissue. The storage of fat in the muscle tissue decreases with age as the binding protein decreases. This means fat from the muscle is less readily available as an energy source during exercise and a greater reliance is placed on other energy stores.
- *increased eating:* Although this is often under-reported, there is evidence to suggest that eating and drinking may actually increase with age, rather than decrease or remain stable, as would be necessary to stabilise body fat.[11] Accurate monitoring of food intake in the elderly will be necessary before this can be verified.

On the positive side, it appears that moderate fat gains with ageing do not appear to be as dangerous as those in the young and a BMI up to $27kg/m^2$ is considered within the normal range for older people. However, this point is still hotly debated and in the meantime caution is still advised.

## OTHER BIOLOGICAL FACTORS

There are some other notable biological factors influencing fat loss which occur at certain periods of life. These include puberty, menses, and menopause and a wide range of genetic factors. Like most biological influences, these are relatively fixed, and hence modifications have generally not been seen as a realistic approach to dealing with the problem. The implications of these biological influences are in accepting factors beyond the control of the obese person. Obesity can no longer be simply ascribed to either 'sloth' or 'gluttony'.

## IMPLICATIONS

1. It is necessary to recognise genetic differences in body shape and composition and the implications of these for fat loss programming.
2. Factors which may indicate a genetic influence in fat loss response (i.e. parental body shape; early onset of overfatness; duration of effect) should be included in any pre-program screening.
3. It may be necessary in certain groups (i.e. the aged, pre-menopausal exercising females) to check the level of spontaneous physical activity being carried out outside a planned exercise regime and attempt to increase this through 'incidental' activity.
4. Individuals with a genetic predisposition to obesity may have difficulty limiting food intake and the taste for fatty foods.
5. Recognise the major gender differences in fat loss responsivity to both energy input restrictions and energy output and design fat loss programs accordingly.
6. Avoid severe restrictions of food intake or heavy exercise prescription in females as these may have a counter-productive effect on the biological propensity of females to conserve energy for reproduction.
7. Recognise the potential for excessive fat gains during and following pregnancy in some women and attempt to offer preventive prescriptions for this, particularly in those most likely to be at risk.
8. Avoid programming which involves unrealistic expectations about body image, particularly in females.
9. Extreme forms of body building with accompanying over-eating disorders in men should be seen as the equivalent of anorexia in females—there are comparative body shape obsessions and distortions.
10. Programming should be modified to account for differences in responses that occur with ageing with both men and women, but particularly in post-menopausal women.
11. Monitor possible changes in eating patterns that occur with ageing, of which the client should be aware.
12. Use body fat and fat distribution measures such as BMI and waist-to-hip ratio cautiously in some racial groups (such as Pacific Islanders, Asian and Negroid women) for whom these measures are not necessarily appropriate.
13. Recognise racial differences in body shape and composition and the implications of this for healthy body weight and fat maintenance.

# 17
# Behavioural influences

SUMMARY OF MAIN POINTS

- The psychological understanding of obesity has moved through several phases in recent times.
- Behaviour modification techniques were initially used widely to change habits.
- Cognitive approaches have been used to change thought patterns.
- Rational Emotive Therapy (RET) is an example of a 'pop' psychology approach to changing thought patterns.
- Other approaches have examined the symbolic nature of fat.
- The task of a fat loss counsellor is complex and involves an understanding of a range of different causalities and interventions.
- Fat loss leaders should develop a close referral link with a qualified psychologist.

The simplistic view of obesity was that if a person ate too much, he or she got fat. The solution was: eat less and you'll lose fat. This is the 'diet as medicine' approach. In reality, the issue is much more complex. Some people couldn't eat less simply as a result of being told; some people could obey the injunction, but could not keep up the practice and some people experienced almost a panic reaction in the face of trying to control their eating. Studying the problem some researchers reported: '. . . it was our feeling that our patients perceived weight reduction, not as a happy end to a disabling disorder, but rather as a threat to the integrity of functioning'.[1] Other research reported not only an increase in depression in overweight people undergoing diets, but also that the same symptoms—increased emotionality, irritability and anxiety—were seen in normal weight people subject to severe food restriction.[2]

## HISTORICAL PERSPECTIVE

The psychological understanding of obesity has moved through several phases;[3] in the 1950s, being too fat was seen by psycho-analysts as deriving from emotional problems—insecurity, anxiety, and repressed sexual needs—which were all represented by over-eating. Research, however, demonstrated that fat people were no more neurotic than thin people, nor was their fatness connected with lower intelligence or educational potential. Fatness does not result from stupidity, although stigmatisation and isolation from peers may lessen the chances of employment or advances in a career.[4] The main personality difference between fat and thin people centres around the former's lowered self-concept and self-image, which are more the consequences of obesity and the social pressures this brings, than any intrinsic cause of obesity.

## BEHAVIOUR MODIFICATION

Behaviour modification became the vogue, based on the theory that fat people are conditioned to eat in response to the 'wrong' stimuli, such as watching TV or being 'bored'. Behavioural mod-ification is centred on the notion that habits are learned patterns of behaviour that usually do not involve complex cognitive, or thinking processes. Change the response and the tendency to eat inappropriately (i.e. in the absence of body hunger signals) or to be inactive, will fade away.

In their simplest form, habits develop as an association between a stimulus and a response. Initially, a stimulus which initiates a response is known as an unconditioned stimulus (US) resulting in an unconditioned response (UR). This stimulus is then paired with a conditioned stimulus (CS) to give a conditioned response (CR). In psychological terms this is known as 'classical conditioning'. Perhaps the best known example is the salivary experiences of Pavlov's dog. Ivan Pavlov was a physiologist living in Russia around the turn of the century. He discovered, not so surprisingly, that every time he presented dinner to his dog, the dog salivated. Pavlov then paired the sound of a bell to the presentation of the food and found, after a while, that the bell alone was all that was necessary to cause the salivation.

---

### MYTH-INFORMATION

*'Spot reduction' (reducing fat by exercising muscle underneath that fat) does not work. Otherwise all gum chewers would have very skinny faces. Fat to power muscle is not necessarily taken from fat sources close to those muscles.*

---

Similar principles can be applied, in a very simplistic way, to humans. An example of a typical learned response to eat in modern society would be getting up from a chair to get something to eat every time an advertisement interrupts a program on television. The association between the advertisement and eating is a surprisingly simple connection, but the kind of thing that people do every day without conscious thought. This is similar to the habits formed in getting dressed, sleeping, working, driving a car, or the myriad of other activities that are carried out automatically during the day.

Examples of eating patterns that are conditioned include:

- eating at the same time every day whether hungry or not
- reading while eating (and thus getting hungry while reading)
- always finishing off everything on the plate
- eating crisps/peanuts with alcohol.

Examples of conditioned inactivity patterns include:

- driving to the shops instead of walking
- getting someone to get something for you rather than getting it yourself
- going for a drink instead of a walk
- sleeping in on cold mornings.

## BREAKING BEHAVIOURAL HABITS

The first stage of any behaviour modification program requires an awareness of the habits that are interfering with a person's goals. This is done by 'stalking one's habits like a hunter stalks his prey'.[5] Once an individual is aware of their CS and CR, it becomes possible to break this stimulus–response connection in a number of different ways (Table 17.1).

Useful information from the behaviour therapy approach includes the conscious modification of eating style through a range of procedures such as those illustrated in Table 17.2.

## CONDITIONS FOR BEHAVIOURAL INTERVENTIONS

Initially, positive results from the behaviour modification approach proved as short lived as other methods of weight control. Although these techniques have value in themselves as part of a wider complex of behavioural interventions, in practice of course, not all behaviours are so simple. In a review of the research on behavioural interventions for weight loss, Stuart asserts that: '. . . the maintenance of weight loss is a mandatory criterion in the evaluation of the behaviour therapy approach'.[6] He concludes that the design of interventions must start with the following assumptions:

1. that obesity is a complex disorder, the culmination of physiological, psychological, social and situational factors;
2. that as a lifestyle disorder, it can only be remedied through a lifetime of effort;
3. that this kind of profound change requires the development of positive alternatives to problem behaviours;
4. that weight loss candidates must address four major stages of weight control: first the decision to commit oneself to action; second, the management of hunger and eating behaviour itself; third, the management of relapse and last, strategies for coping with long term maintenance.

## CHANGING COGNITIVE PATTERNS

Following this, more sophisticated approaches have been developed incorporating cognitive behavioural techniques, more realistic

**Table 17.1: Processes for modifying stimulus response connections**

1. Monitoring
2. Changing the stimulus
3. Changing the response
4. Changing the stimulus–response connection

**Table 17.2: Behaviour modification approaches for modifying eating style**

| Cue elimination and physical environment | Manner of eating | Food choice | Alternative activities |
|---|---|---|---|
| Eat only in designated place | Slow rate of eating—chew slowly | Portion control—cut snacks in half | Exercise—walking or jogging, other aerobic activities, recreational activities |
| Eat only when sitting in designated place | Swallow each bite before taking a second one | Measure foods until portions can be estimated | Relaxation |
| Set regular eating times | Put utensils down between bites | Serve only amounts planned | Meditation |
| Plan snacks and meals ahead | Count mouthfuls | Preplan eating when entertaining; set aside portions | Imagery (visualise foods to be in an inedible form or think of being in another place) |
| Determine degree of hunger before eating | Pause in the middle of a meal for a few minutes | Share dessert | Do necessary tasks, errands, yard work, or housework |
| Dissociate eating from other activities (e.g., reading, watching television) | Relax 60 seconds before eating | Include favourite foods | Write a letter |
| Plan and order restaurant meals ahead | Savour foods; enjoy each bite | Eat a variety of foods | Call someone |
| Store all foods; use opaque containers or store in inaccessible places | Eat only until reaching a 'satisfied' hunger level (not until 'stuffed') | Have appropriate snacks planned and 'ready to go' | Do problem solving |
| Use small plates and bowls | Allow at least 20 minutes for eating a meal | Serve 'on-the-side' dressings and sauces | Re-evaluate goals and priorities |
| Let others get their snacks | Leave 5% to 20% of meal uneaten | Use spices instead of high-calorie condiments | Practice assertiveness |
| Record food intake | Push food aside ahead of time | Use garnishes (attractive and take up space on the plate) | Make charts for progress |
| Shop when not hungry, and use a list | Cover plate with napkin when finished eating | Use low-calorie ingredient substitutes | Take up a reward for following plans |
| Store foods out of sight | | | Brush teeth |
| Avoid 'problem' places and people | | | Take a bath or shower |
| Serve buffets | | | Go for a drive |
| Remove plate from eating place after meal | | | |
| Clean plates directly into garbage | | | |
| Change route of travel to bypass a tempting eating place | | | |
| Write notes as reminders or use pictures; put on mirrors or refrigerator | | | |

*Source:* O'Donnell, M., and Ainsworth, T. *Health promotion in the workplace*. Philadelphia: John Wiley & Sons, 1984, pp. 312–313. Used with permission goal setting, and a focus on dealing with relapses—by prevention as well as psychological reframing.

Cognitions, such as negative thinking patterns, can be more complex and much more difficult to deal with than simple behavioural habits. People can often give the appearance of smoothly gliding through life with very few complications, while underneath being deep in turmoil. There are a range of ways psychologists deal with this from psychoanalysis to group therapies. Many modern psychological practices, however, now recognise that it is *thinking* about what *may* happen as much as what *actually has* or *is about* to happen, that causes many pathologies, phobias and simple unconstructive behaviours. This is not new. Indeed, there are a range of historical quotations dating back to 500BC which suggest that this is the case (Table 17.3). These provide a clue as to the appropriate means of dealing with major cognitive problems.

## RATIONAL EMOTIVE THERAPY

In many cases, our thought patterns have been programmed by life, coming from inter-personal relationships, childhood experiences or situations of emotional trauma. The extent to which the fat loss leader needs to recognise and deal with these is covered more extensively in separate publications.[7] An introductory perspective, however, can be gained from some of the more popular psychological techniques. Rational Emotive Therapy (RET) is an example of one of these. Developed by US psychologist Albert Ellis[8] in the 1950s, this technique has now been adopted by many modern popular psychologists including Chicago University's Professor Martin Seligman. Seligman is a psychologist who discovered, when working with animals in the 1960s and 1970s, that living organisms can have a tendency to defeatism if continually placed in powerless situations. If a rat is constantly shocked, for example, with no escape available, it eventually gives up and settles down to its fate, which is often death. Similarly, in very deprived circumstances, human beings learn helplessness—they actually regard their situation as hopeless and don't even try.

Seligman called this experience 'learned helplessness' and published a book on the topic in 1974.[9] After a 20-year gap he then published what he considered to be the antidote to this, 'learned optimism'[10] in which he utilises a lot of the techniques used by Albert Ellis in RET. Ellis' approach was developed to

**Table 17.3: The significance of thought patterns in behaviour**

*'We are a result of everything we have thought'*
                          Gautama Siddhartha (the Buddha) 500BC

*'People are disturbed not by things, but by the views they take of them'*
                          Epictetus, 50AD

*'There's nothing either good or bad but thinking makes it so'.*
                          Shakespeare—*Hamlet*

*'I am that which must be overcome'*
                          Friedrich Nietzsche

*'My life has been full of catastrophes, most of which have never happened.'*
                          Mark Twain

counteract his own shyness as a young psychology student and his inability to communicate because of this. He reasoned that this inability was because of the anticipated anxiety he felt every time he went to make contact with another individual (in Mark Twain's terms his life was full of *'potential disasters'*). Ellis realised that the problem was within himself, because of the way he *thought* about the situation; it was his *belief* that he was an unworthy person, because he *must* always succeed, other people *must* always treat him well and the world *must* be good to him. He realised, however, that these beliefs were *irrational*, and based on no solid, objective evidence. In a similar way, it is the belief of many fat people, that they are unworthy and that others regard them as unworthy, while in reality, others are generally too concerned about their own problems to even consider them. This belief can then become self-fulfilling, exacerbating the problem of overfatness itself.

Ellis based his thesis of RET around a very simple format based on the letters ABCD (Figure 17.1).

Ellis claimed: 'We consciously and unconsciously choose to think and hence to feel in certain self-helping and self-harming ways' and 'Once you understand the basic irrational beliefs you create to upset yourself, you can use this understanding to explore, attack, and surrender your other present and future emotional problems'.

As you can see in Figure 17.1, there is an A, or *Adversity*, which generally starts the rot. In the case of a fat person trying to maintain an extreme diet or exercise regime, this might be a situation which breaks the pattern, such as a binge, or over-eating session. Adversity then, according to Ellis, usually takes a jump, leading to C or the *Consequence* of this adversity. By bingeing, the fat person may then think, *'I'm worthless; I can never do anything right; it could only happen to me'*. However, it is the

**Figure 17.1: The ABCD approach to rational emotive therapy**

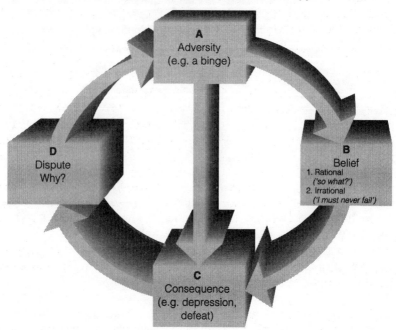

jump here from A to C which results in this form of thinking and which may lead to resignation and relapse.

Weight cycling, resulting from binge eating then dieting, is a common phenomenon with potential influences from this kind of thought process.[11] Up to 50 per cent of females and 16 per cent of males who are dieters are of normal weight.[12] While some degree of restrained eating to prevent weight gain might be included in these figures, they are sufficiently high to imply an irrationality of cognitive processes perhaps instigated by unrealistic social pressures. As can be seen from Figure 17.1, it is the intermediary process or B, for *Beliefs*, which are the real cause of much of these *Consequences*. It is a person's irrational belief that s/he *must* always be perfect and *must* never stray, that leads to unproductive outcomes, not the actuality of the situation itself. It is these beliefs which may ultimately lead to self-defeat in the behaviour of that individual.

Beliefs, according to Ellis, can be *rational* or *irrational*. Irrational beliefs which, according to Ellis are the major problem in maladaptive behaviours, are generally associated with *musts*, *shoulds* and *have to's*, and are usually 'hot', or charged with emotion in comparison with rational beliefs which are more 'cool' or 'warm'. An example of an irrational belief would be 'I MUST NEVER binge or I am a bad person', or 'I HAVE TO always be good or I will feel miserable and horrible'.

It is easy to see how these irrational beliefs can lead one into cognitive habits, or thinking patterns, that are self-defeating, self-limiting and self-punishing. Ellis, therefore, adds D or Disputation to his program in order to help overcome these irrational beliefs. An individual should learn to systematically analyse his or her beliefs, he claims, and logically argue against these. This cannot be done by the therapist, but it may be aided. For example, the question can be asked: '*Why must you always succeed on your diet or eating plan? It may be nice, but must it always happen? What would be the worst consequence if this did not happen? Could you live with this? What are the consequences of maintaining this irrational approach?*' The thought process is thus 'reframed' to provide an opportunity to reduce irrational thoughts.

Ellis regards '*mus*turbation' as one of the main problems of psychopathology. He considers there are three main types of overpowering 'musts' i.e.:

1. I MUST always be perfect.
2. You MUST treat me well, or you are an awful person.
3. The world MUST always be good to me or it is a horrible place.

There are also ten common forms of irrational beliefs that are self-limiting in this sense. These, and some examples of them relating to body fat maintenance, are listed in Table 17.4.

RET is a relatively simplistic approach to a complex problem. It is used for a range of different psychopathologies including fear

**Table 17.4: Ten common forms of irrational thinking relating to body fat maintenance**

1. All or nothing ('*If I don't starve myself I'll get fat*')
2. Over-generalisation ('*Things always go wrong*')
3. Mental filter ('*It's not the program, it's me thats wrong*')
4. Disqualifying the positive ('*That was just luck*')
5. Jumping to conclusions:
   (a) mind reading ('*S/he thinks I'm useless*')
   (b) fortune telling ('*If I did lose fat, he wouldn't like me*')
6. Catastrophising ('*The world will end tomorrow if I fail*')
7. Emotional reasoning ('*I feel so upset because I'm a failure*')
8. Musturbating ('*I must never eat anything fattening*')
9. Labelling ('*I'm a loser*')
10. The 3 P's: personal, permanent and pervasive ('*It only happens to me: I'll always be like this: It's the same with everything I do*')

*Source:* Adapted from Ellis (1975)[8]

251

of flying, fear of spiders and many other phobias. It has potential use in body fat maintenance, although it would not be expected to be applicable under all circumstances. In many instances, such as those that lead to problems of obesity, there may be a role for a more detailed approach to the problem.

## OTHER APPROACHES

The late 1970s saw a shift towards portraying fat as a symbol in a person's life, particularly in the lives of women, and a re-examination of the psychodynamic aspects of being overfat. Susie Orbach saw fat as a kind of defensive psychological smoke screen, an unconscious rebellion for a woman against her sense of powerlessness in society.[13] Compulsive eating, then, not only serves the deeper purpose of maintaining the distance between her real self and the rest of the world, but also acts to 'blot out' unacceptable feelings and thoughts. The problems of fatness become a reflection of a woman's cultural position of inferiority; her compulsion to control her eating as a displacement of her inability to deal with other more profound aspects of her life. This theme was then taken up and expanded by Naomi Wolfe who sees the apparent epidemic in eating disorders as symbolic of society's need to keep increasingly educated young women in a state of semi-starvation, rendering them 'no trouble'.[14]

Obviously this approach requires a different response to the behavioural strategies discussed above; if eating problems are caused by an existential and societal inequality, addressing the issue of powerlessness becomes the theme of both group and individual therapy. However, it is unclear from the feminist perspective how to account for the large numbers of men who acquire excessive fat. Presumably it is not for the same reasons of frustration and powerlessness, nor that they need to be assisted to come to terms with their 'real' selves. Perhaps males more easily fall into the trap of the 'unconscious' habits which more readily respond to the behaviour modification approaches. It seems highly likely that strategies need to be tailored to suit the individual.

## THE PSYCHOLOGICAL COMPLEXITY OF OBESITY

The complexity of psychological factors involved in obesity is shown in the 4 phases of weight loss and regain shown in Figure 17.2.

**Figure 17.2: A model of psychological components in weight loss and regain**

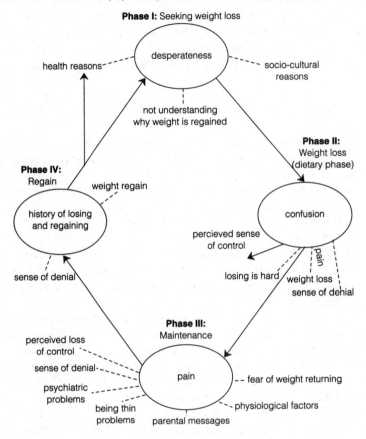

*Source:* Wysoker (1994)[15]

Feeling pressured to be lean, a fat person may starve him or herself, which in the long run is self-defeating and biologically impossible to sustain. S/he will then eat (perhaps a lot), but feel guilty for doing so. Guilt leads to depression, and one of the early refuges for depression is food. So depression leads to eating—and the cycle continues.

## THE TASK OF THE FAT LOSS COUNSELLOR

The following lists some basic tasks and resources which can be used by the fat loss counsellor in exploring the psychological component of excess body fatness.[15] More detailed therapy should be referred to a qualified professional psychologist.

## Current attitudes

1. Identify current thoughts, feelings and attitudes to fat loss: What for? Why now? How long for? What then? Ensure clients recognise that permanent fat loss means lifestyle change.
2. Clarify expectations of fat loss: What problems are anticipated that it will solve? How else could these problems be dealt with? If any of these expectations are perceived negatively, how else could the problem be managed?
3. Clearly define a lifestyle which is both acceptable and achievable, which will maintain a lower level of both fat intake and body fat level.

## History

1. Explore previous experiences of fat/weight loss: What worked, What didn't? What lasted? How were relapses dealt with? Understand what went wrong or right and how this time is different.
2. Deal with family 'leftovers', experience of fatness in the family, food messages, how eating, drinking and exercise played a part in the family life and what impact these still have.

## Obstacles

1. Identify which important aspects of lifestyle keep the client from losing fat: food choices, feelings/experiences which seem associated with inappropriate eating, time pressure, stress, lack of regular exercise, food knowledge?
2. Identify times during the day/week which represent the most difficult times to control eating: Mealtimes? Snack times? Going to work? Going home? Eating out?

## Knowledge

1. How good is the client's knowledge of what is in food? How is this used? What else is happening at times when fattier food is deliberately chosen?
2. Increase knowledge of low-fat shopping, cooking, recipe modification and food skills associated with developing palatable, low-fat foods.

*Possible resources:* Health Department; National Heart Foundation; nutrition organisations.

### Stress management

1. Identify possible connections between perceived stress and eating behaviour.
2. Develop effective stress management techniques which do not involve the use of food, in conjunction with other regularly used 'self-nourishing' activities.
3. Plan and use time consistent with lifestyle aims (i.e. incorporating deliberate and incidental exercise, food choices and meal planning).
4. Develop and practice assertiveness, with self and others.

*Possible resources*: Stress management courses; psychological therapy; meditation, relaxation courses.

### Habit management

1. 'Reframe' eating habits which contribute to overfatness as 'curious and interesting' as opposed to 'immoral or bad'.
2. 'Stalk'—describe eating, drinking, exercise avoidance habits or routines and develop strategies for interrupting these. Monitor self-talk, identify triggers for over-eating and thinking patterns associated with these. Challenge beliefs about self body image.
3. Evaluate social environment for social support. Develop ways to protect self from 'high risk' situations.

*Possible resources:* Psychological therapy; behaviour therapy; community health centres.

### Relapse management

1. Identify and develop a clear strategy for dealing with relapses. This includes strategies for dealing with celebrations and festivities, times of high stress and pressure, times of boredom alone and negative mood states.

### Sometimes a client just doesn't lose weight—why not?

Below are frequently stated items that often require psychological counselling to resolve. These issues are not, in themselves, the reason why a person is fat, but they may serve to maintain a level of overfatness by acting as the psychological trigger for inappropriate eating, may impair the individual's ability to cope with stress, and may leave him or her vulnerable as adults, especially in the face of plentiful food supplies.

1. Unresolved food or eating issues from the client's family:
   - the use or withholding of food to punish, humiliate or isolate
   - the frequent use of food as a reward for 'being good', 'being quiet', 'stopping crying' or 'being brave'
   - unfair treatment by one or several family members associated with food or inequality or competition in its distribution (e.g. 'if I didn't eat my share there and then my brother would get it')
   - the production or consumption of food to show affection, appreciation or avoid a confrontation
   - pressure to eat: repeated messages such as 'clean up your plate or you'll get sick'; 'finish your main course or you won't get dessert'; 'think of all the starving children in . . . (insert third world country)'
   - a form of 'toxic parenting' associated with low levels of care combined with high levels of control.
2. Previous trauma such as:
   - childhood, teenage or adult sexual or physical abuse
   - periods of acute starvation, including those self-induced (e.g. anorexia)
   - mental abuse, especially associated with body image
   - unexpected birth trauma and/or postnatal depression associated with weight gain.

MYTH-INFORMATION
*The suggestion that all obesity and overfatness problems have a biological origin ignores the complexity of human behaviour. Past experience as well as thought patterns and habits are significant factors in causing and maintaining excessive body fat.*

3. Current problems with partner(s) and/or family:
   - marital problems which involve a partner's perception of body shape, looks or pressure to be thin
   - fear of sexuality
   - continued influence or control from family on eating habits and body shape/size
   - assumption that the lack of a partner is associated with being fat.
4. Lifestyle problems:
   - stress
   - over-commitment and poor time management
   - high priority on work status and low priority on health status
   - being 'stuck' in a situation which may not be of one's own choice, e.g. as a 'carer'.
5. Low self-esteem accompanied by:
   - frequent use of high-fat/sugar foods to comfort or alleviate distress
   - little use of other self-nourishing behaviours
   - negative self and body image, punitive internal dialogue
   - use of food both to reward and punish self
   - deletion or distortion of much positive feedback, verbal and non-verbal
   - tendency towards negative self-fulfilling prophecies
   - frequently feeling 'like a victim'
   - perfectionist standards for both self and others (all-or-nothing)
   - lack of assertive skills
   - tendency to depression
   - the feeling of not being entitled to eat.

**Knowing when to refer on**

Clients should be referred on to a specialist psychologist or psychiatric services when any of the following indicators are present:

- A client is clearly very distressed by his or her eating problems
- He or she is locked into a rigid regime of exercise and/or eating patterns and gets disturbed by any disruption to these

- Laxatives or vomiting is used to control weight
- They talk to you about thoughts of suicide
- There is a history of sexual or physical abuse
- They report other stress related symptoms such as sleep problems, feeling out of control or depressed
- There is a need for grief or depression counselling.

## IMPLICATIONS

1. The purpose of counselling is to empower clients so that they can develop an awareness of their habits, prioritise those things to work on and be selective about those techniques most appropriate for the task.
2. Fat loss leaders need to develop a close liaison with professional psychologists for referring complex cases.
3. In dealing with habits, the first stage is to develop an awareness of the components of the habit.
4. There is a range of techniques for changing behavioural habit patterns including interrupting stimulus–response connections, changing the stimulus, reinforcement and self-monitoring. Not all techniques work for all people.
5. Negative thinking habits can be worked on using standard psychological techniques such as rational emotive therapy, positive thinking, etc.
6. Behaviour modification and cognitive therapy techniques need to be maintained over the long term and not just used in the initial stages of fat loss. This takes longer than most people anticipate and a realistic expectation is important.
7. It should be assumed that the majority, if not all, overfat problems require at least a modicum of change in habit patterns. The degree to which this is so and the types of approaches used to combat these will depend on the individual and the circumstances.

# IX
# OTHER ISSUES

# 18

# Critical periods for fat gain and relapse

### SUMMARY OF MAIN POINTS

- There are a number of critical periods throughout life where gains and losses in body fat and body weight are likely to occur.
- Some of these are due to physiological causes, others to behaviour and/or periods of high stress, crisis or grief.
- Restrained eaters may be likely to gain more fat during periods of chronic stress, crisis or grief.
- Awareness of critical stages and actions that can be taken to resolve these may help prevent or reduce increases in body fatness.

Although the causes of obesity and overfatness are multi-factorial, the problem may be exacerbated at certain critical' periods in life. These are generally associated with *change*, either in lifestyle, as a result of crises or increased levels of stress, or due to the natural physiological changes that occur with ageing. As some psychologists have pointed out, change is often associated with increased stress levels, even in some cases where these changes are positive. Stress, in turn, can be crucial for either increasing or decreasing body fat depending on the circumstances. There are periods that predominantly affect either males or females and others that are less gender specific. Some are potentially avoidable and others are an unavoidable function of the ongoing processes of growth and

**Table 18.1: Critical periods for fat gain and relapse**

| Influences | Critical period |
|---|---|
| Hormonal | Adolescence |
| | Pregnancy |
| | Menopause |
| Stress and anxiety | Prolonged stress |
| | Grief/bereavement |
| | Divorce/separation |
| Lifestyle related changes | Retirement from sport |
| | Marriage |
| | Middle age in men |
| | Festive occasions |
| Physiological | Quitting smoking |
| | After weight loss |
| | Due to some medications |

change. An awareness of at least some of these critical periods and the potential means of alleviating their effects is crucial to an understanding of long term body fat maintenance. Although the scientific evidence on some of the periods shown in Table 18.1 is limited, practical suggestions based on experience are discussed for each period.

## HORMONAL CHANGES

### Adolescence

It is now thought that excess hyperplasia of fat cells is possible during periods of rapid growth when all body cells proliferate.[1] One particular stage for this is the early adolescent period, around 12–14 years of age. Adolescents who are inactive at this stage and/or eating high energy foods, may develop more fat cells and then retain these for life. Crash dieting and binges that are common in adolescent girls may exacerbate the problem by setting patterns for fatness and may be one reason for long term obesity problems.

Physical activity at this stage of life is vital. Excessive TV viewing in adolescents has been linked with inactivity which may foreshadow the development of obesity in an adult.[2] Prevention strategies at this critical period are obviously preferable and easier than trying to cure overfatness later in life. More recognition needs to be given to this fact in public health approaches to the problem.

One prominent study carried out in the US has shown that strategies which decrease TV viewing and other inactive pastimes may be more effective as a fat loss technique in children than

━━━━━━━━━━━━━━━━━━━━━━━━━━━━━━━━━━

MYTH-INFORMATION
*Any fat loss program that proclaims 'no exercise, no effort' needs to be looked at suspiciously. While it is possible to lose fat through diet alone, long term maintenance of fat loss requires at least a moderate level of physical activity.*

━━━━━━━━━━━━━━━━━━━━━━━━━━━━━━━━━━

attempting to increase their involvement in physical activity and sports.[3]

## Pregnancy

Pregnancy and body weight increases are intertwined in a complicated pattern. Female fat stores have a primary function to provide energy for pregnancy and lactation. A pregnant woman requires approximately 130 000 kcal extra as the metabolic cost of pregnancy.[4] Women who tend to put on too much fat in the early stages of pregnancy have been shown to keep this longer than those who do not put on excessive fat, or put on most fat later in the pregnancy. The recommended weight gain during pregnancy by the US medical specialists has risen from 7–8kg in the 1920s to 10–12kg in the 1970s. In 1989, the National Task Force on Prevention and Treatment of Obesity raised the recommendations to 14–16kg in 1995. However, there are now suggestions by some experts that this is too much and that the most recent recommendations are based simply on the modern average weight gain of pregnant women in the US. The previously recommended gain of 10–12kg has been suggested as a more appropriate health ideal for which to aim.[5]

Breast-feeding is also known to be an effective form of fat burning, using up to 400kcal of energy per day.[6] In one study carried out in the US, women who breast-fed for at least six months stayed leaner for up to two years than women who did not breast-feed at all or did so for less than six months.[7] It has also been claimed that the risk of obesity increases with parity or the number of childbirths. This may be due to the repetitive exposure to the fat storing hormones of pregnancy, restrictions on physical activity or increased opportunity to eat more. In any case, for some women, pregnancy does appear to be a particularly high risk period for increases in obesity.

Research from the Stockholm Pregnancy and Weight Development Study in Sweden[8] suggests that the greater the weight gain during pregnancy, the more likely the increase in post-partum body fat levels. Cessation of smoking with the onset of pregnancy may increase weight gain in the mother (although it certainly reduces the risk of birth complications in the baby). Those women who gained most weight during and after pregnancy were found to be those who had significantly changed their lifestyle from pre-pregnancy levels such as increased eating/snack eating and decreased levels of physical activity. Maintenance of physical activity through pregnancy and attention to nutrition, therefore, are most important to ensure a return to normal fat levels, but there are also special considerations for exercise which need to be considered. These are now available from most Health Departments.

## Menopause

Changes in hormonal status in females around menopause mean that there are likely to be changes in body composition.[9] Post-menopausal females are likely to become more apple shaped, like males, but in many cases still maintain their body fat content around the hips and thighs. As with males, upper body fat is relatively more lipolytic and therefore responds easier to standard fat loss procedures in post-menopausal women. Hence, upper body fat loss should be no more difficult than for males, unlike the lower body fat stores of pre-menopausal women. It should be remembered, however, that there are natural decreases in metabolic rate with age and a tendency for older people to be less active and to eat more as they age. These changes need to be actively countered to prevent excessive fat gain in this stage of life.

Maintenance of muscle mass with the addition of some resistance training can help to reduce the impact of menopause.[10] The use of hormone replacement therapy (HRT) may also be useful for body composition maintenance in the post-menopausal period, although the type of hormonal mix and other factors may also play a part (see below).

### STRESS AND ANXIETY

## Chronic stress

There is good anecdotal evidence of a link between stress and body fat levels, although the association is a complex one. Under cases of acute, life threatening stress, animals (including humans) stop eating and go into a protection mode. They also tend to burn more energy, both through increased physical activity and increased 'nervous energy'. However, most modern day stress is usually less life threatening and more chronic, or long term in nature. Under these circumstances many humans—particularly fat ones—tend to eat more, drink more alcohol, and generally become less active, all factors predisposing to increases in body fatness.

Long term, 'chronic' stress can increase obesity by:

- encouraging over-eating (especially of high-fat snack foods)
- immobilising efforts to improve lifestyle
- decreasing feelings of 'self control'
- decreasing self-esteem
- consuming available energy and efforts while in survival mode
- increasing alcohol consumption.

'Restrained eaters' (those who restrict their food intake because of consciousness of being too fat) tend to be most likely to gain fat under periods of chronic stress.[11] Caution about eating, and all other concerns about food intake usually go by the wayside with long term increases in stress levels and food may serve a 'comfort' role to the stressed individual. In one research study, women were shown to be more prone to over-eating during stressful periods, whereas only men regarded as 'emotional eaters' respond in this way.[12] In any case, anyone prone to fat gain during stressful situations should perhaps deal with the stress as a means of body fat regulation. Stress alleviation initiatives, therefore, may be an integral part of a body fat management program for some individuals.

**Grief, bereavement and depression**

Grief, bereavement and/or depression are periods of distress for most people during which the normal restraints required for fat control become regarded as less important in the same way as they are in periods of chronic stress (above). Again, these are times during which physical activity can be expected to decrease and eating, particularly of 'comfort foods', increase. Depending on the circumstances, these periods can last for anything from days to several years. Additional stressors on top of the initial bereavement might then add to the problem.

Predicting those who may gain or lose fat as a result of depression is not a simple task. In a study carried out by the US

National Health and Nutrition Examination Survey (NHANES)[13] it was found that younger men (less than 55 years of age) who were depressed seemed to put on more weight over time than those who were not. This was particularly so if education levels were low. In contrast, depressed young women seemed to put on less weight than their non-depressed counterparts. But again, education levels seemed to play a part with the more highly educated putting on less weight with depression than those with lesser education. In these instances, psychological counselling to deal with grief and depression should be the primary process of any intervention rather than initiatives dealing with obesity *per se*.

### Divorce or separation

Like bereavement, divorce or separation has the potential for great psychological disruption to an individual's life. Again, during this time, lifestyle requirements suffer as the need for health sinks lower in an individual's hierarchy of needs. Again, the primary concern is to deal with the psychological anguish associated with the primary cause rather than attempt to impose yet another stressor on the individual. There are some indications that women cope with divorce or separation better than men. Because they often have better coping skills, it might be predicted, therefore, that a woman's gain in body fatness after these periods may be less than that of a man's, although there is little scientific evidence to support this.

MYTH-INFORMATION
*'Fat-burning' tablets are a figment of the marketers' imagination. No tablets (especially those sold without prescription) will have a permanent, long term effect on fat loss, and many can be counter-productive.*

## LIFESTYLE RELATED CHANGES

### Marriage

Marriage, or its equivalent, is often a time where both partners tend to gain fatness and decrease fitness together. Research carried out at the University of Sydney shows that this is particularly so for young males, possibly due to a decreased level of physical activity as their involvement in organised sport drops off, and increased regular food intake.[14] Other studies carried out in the US suggest that it is females who increase weight most, particularly in the short term after marriage.[15] The differences are likely to depend on the circumstances, but either way it is important at this stage to ensure that physical activity is maintained and that there is not an excessive increase in intake of energy dense fatty foods during this period.

## Middle age in males

Decreases in resting metabolic rate (RMR), which occur at around the rate of 2 per cent per decade from age 20, start to have a significant impact with males at around 40–50 years of age.[16] It is at this time that men's rate of physical activity also tends to decline and consumption of food and drink tends to increase. The male 'middle-age spread' carries a substantial increased disease risk. Because abdominal fat is metabolically active, a return to normal levels of body fat is not difficult for most men under the appropriate conditions.[17] An awareness of the 'natural' body fat gains which occur with age can help to alleviate guilt and depression often associated with this.

## During festive occasions

It's well-known that the worst time of the year for the sale of weight control programs is the period leading up to the festive season at Christmas. The best time, on the other hand, is immediately after New Year. For most people, festive periods— including Christmas, Easter, birthdays, re-unions and other cultural and individual celebrations—are a time when enjoyment is likely to over-rule moderation. The occasion is thus often used as a justification for indulgence, with a view to 'making up for this' at some later stage. From a practical perspective, it is probably more appropriate to try to ensure there are no gains in body fat—even if there are no losses—during these periods! If maintenance can ensure stability, it becomes more feasible, both psychologically and physiologically, to continue with improvements at a later stage.

## Retirement from sport

Organised sport can be a motivator for regular physical activity. In the case of top level sports such as the football codes, the level of activity required for performance is high, with training sometimes occurring for 1–3 hours per day, 6–7 days a week. A high energy intake is necessary to fuel this increased energy output. Eating at this rate could then be expected to become a habit (e.g. meals mean 2–3 big helpings; daytime cues such as time of the day can often condition an eating response, the body becomes used to late evening snacks). Retirement from sporting activity often takes place suddenly, with a drastic decrease in energy levels. If there is a maintenance of energy intake, increases in body fatness might be expected. De-conditioning is, therefore, needed at sports retirement with extra education for the retiring athlete. This has currently become part of the employment package of some US professional sporting codes and is likely to be more so in the future, as clubs face greater prospects of litigation. Meanwhile, a decrease in sporting involvement should be seen as a potential risk factor for increases in body fatness calling for increases in compensatory activity levels, or education based around decreased energy input.

## PHYSIOLOGICAL

## After quitting smoking

Smokers who quit have been shown to gain an average of around 3.5kg of body *weight* over twelve months after quitting. This is due to a variety of reasons. Nicotine tends to speed up metabolic rate and a significant drop is noted on quitting. Smoking also suppresses the taste and smell senses so that after smoking cessation, food can smell and taste better. Also, withdrawal from nicotine is a difficult experience and activities involving the hands and mouth (such as eating) are often used as a substitute for smoking.

Research carried out at the University of California, however, has shown that not all quitting smokers put on weight.[18] There are those who gain a lot (over 12kg), those who gain a little (up to 3kg), those whose weight remains stable, and those who actually lose weight. In over 2000 twins studied over 16 years, the percentages in each category were as shown in Table 18.2.

**Table 18.2: Proportion of quitting smokers who gain, lose or maintain weight**

|  | Quitters | Non-smokers | Continuing smokers |
|---|---|---|---|
| Super-gainers | 13% | 4% | 6% |
| Gainers | 39% | 30% | 29% |
| Weight stable | 33% | 45% | 42% |
| Weight losers | 15% | 21% | 23% |

Source:   Swan, G.E. & Carmelli, D. (1995)[16]

Comparisons of super-gainers with non-gainers after quitting showed that super-gainers were younger, of lower socioeconomic status, started smoking at a younger age, were heavier smokers, exercised less and drank more coffee than non-gainers. There were no differences in their body mass before quitting, the number of alcoholic drinks taken per month, or the likelihood of dieting to keep weight low. Hence, lifestyle and socioeconomic factors seem to influence whether there is weight gain or not after smoking.

Interestingly, comparisons between identical and non identical twins showed that there was considerable similarity in weight change after quitting amongst the identical twins. This suggests genetic factors may also be important in determining whether weight gain occurs after quitting smoking.

## After weight loss

Preventing a regain after fat loss is a major challenge especially in people with a genetic predisposition to obesity. As discussed in Chapter 14, there is marked adaptation to fat losses generally regarded as fat loss plateaus. These may also correspond with changes in psychological factors including depression at not having achieved the losses expected.

Currently, there is little written about plateaus and little specific research in the area, even though this is one of the most critical concepts in fat loss maintenance. It is generally because of a plateau in fat loss, and the inability to do anything about this, that disillusionment sets in and a program is abandoned.

The length of time spent on plateaus is variable and appears to have individual idiosyncrasies. In general, the time period *increases* with the extent of initial fat loss. The magnitude of the fat loss off a plateau on the other hand *decreases* the greater the fat loss from the initial level (see Figure 18.1). Plateaus, as well as overall fat mass decreases, also appear to be a function of the length of time an individual has been overfat or obese. It thus becomes more difficult to lose fat over the long term, the longer

**Figure 18.1: Rate of fat loss and fat loss plateaus over time**

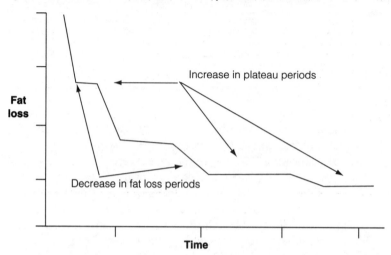

one has been fat in the first place and the longer a maintenance program needs to be carried out. Figures 18.1 and 18.2 show this schematically.

In Figure 18.1, the length of plateaus is shown to increase and the rate of fat loss is shown to decline with increased loss, basically as a result of the adaptive mechanisms referred to earlier.

In Figure 18.2, the postulated differences in the responses to slimming between a long term obese and short term overfat person are shown. Note how the plateaus are likely to be longer and the rates of fat loss smaller in the long term obese than the short term overfat person.

It is important for anyone on a fat loss program to recognise that plateaus are inevitable stages that occur in the maintenance of fat loss. It's necessary, therefore, for any professional working in the area to communicate that provided there is no *increase* in body fat during these periods (as there is likely to be due to disillusionment with the lack of success), they should be tolerated. A general principle is that '. . . *as long as you're not gaining, you're winning!'* Plateaus should be regarded as the body 'taking a breather' to ensure it can survive under reduced energy balance.

## Breaking through plateaus

The first process in dealing with plateaus is an acceptance of the fact that this is a normal and natural process. Provided there is

**Figure 18.2: The effects of duration of obesity on adaptations to slimming**

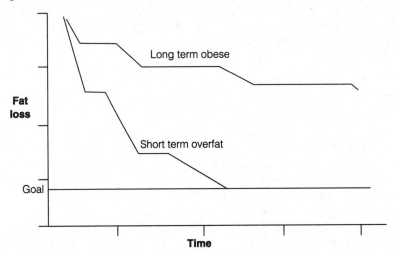

no increase in fat mass, the plateau can be countered by attacking the causes. Dietary and exercise habits should be revisited and physiological adaptations to change can, at least theoretically, be 'shocked' into change. In terms of exercise load this will mean making physical activity *less efficient* by changing:

* intensity—increase the speed a regular movement is carried out
* duration—carry out the exercise for longer periods
* frequency—move more regularly (e.g. by adding 'incidental' exercise)
* type—vary walking with cycling, swimming, aerobics etc.

With food intake as the other side of the energy equation, plateaus might be countered by:

* decreasing energy intake—but only where this is still high
* increasing energy intake—by re-feeding where intake is excessively low (i.e. under 1000 kcal/day), and has been so for long periods
* decreasing fat intake further
* reducing alcohol intake
* changing food type—eating foods with which the body may not be familiar.[19]

These changes might help an individual break through a plateau then restart and continue reducing fat. The introduction of resistance training as a form of exercise at this stage of a

271

program may also be useful (if desired by the client), not only because of its 'shock' value, but also because of the potential maintenance of lean body tissue which can help counteract the physiological adaptations leading to plateauing.

### Disillusionment

Disillusionment is a psychological phenomenon that is also characteristic of the maintenance phase of fat loss. Whilst anyone starting a program seriously is likely to be highly motivated, this can change as a result of a number of different factors. Plateaus, in particular, can cause disillusionment and lead someone to want to give it all away. Other things like short binges, holiday seasons, re-unions with friends, and critical periods in life can also cause the disillusionment which is the curse of those wishing to lose fat. When disillusionment and plateaus coincide, extra psychological principles are needed to help individuals get through this stage.

## Prescribed medications

There are a number of medications, including those prescribed for anxiety, depression, schizophrenia and inflammatory conditions,[20] that affect body fat stores. A list of drugs known to either increase body fat or make it more difficult to lose fat is shown in Table 18.3. Most of these affect body fat levels by either stimulating appetite or decreasing energy use through changes in central nervous system function. Androgens may increase body *weight* through increased fluid retention and increased muscular bulk.

### STRATEGIES TO PREVENT RELAPSE

Many of the changes discussed above that occur over the longer term with slimming make relapse a key issue in fat loss maintenance. Long term studies (i.e. over 10 years) show that the cure rate for obesity is usually no more than 5–10 per cent.[21] Even 1–2 year follow-ups with females show a high attrition rate (i.e. 40–60 per cent) and the success rate for males is largely unknown. About 80 per cent of people who go on a fat loss program can lose 10–20 per cent of their weight in up to 20 weeks without too much pain. However, within 12 months, about one-third of those who have lost fat will have regained it. The problem is even worse for those following a very low energy diet. Regain occurs

**Table 18.3: Prescribed medications which may affect fat or weight loss**

*Androgens (male hormones)*

| *Generic name:* | *Brand name:* |
|---|---|
| ethyloestrenol | Orabolin |
| fluroxymesterone | Halotestin |
| nandrolone | Durabolin |
| oxymetholone | Adroyd |
| stanozolol | Winstrol |
| testosterone | Andriol |
| | Primoteston |
| | Sustanon |

*Benzodiazapines (anti-anxiety)*

| *Generic name:* | *Brand name:* |
|---|---|
| (a) | |
| alprozolam | Xanax |
| chlordiazepoxide | Librium |
| clorozepate | Tranxene |
| diazepam | Valium |
| lorazepam | Ativan |
| oxazepam | Serapax |
| (b) | |
| flurazepam | Dalmane |
| temazepam | Normison |
| triazolam | Halcion |
| nitrazepam | Mogadon |

*Corticosteroids (anti-allergy; anti-inflammatory)*

| *Generic name:* | *Brand name:* |
|---|---|
| (a) | |
| betamethasone | Celestone |
| dexamethasone | Decadron |
| methylprednisolone | Medrol |
| prednisolone | Delta-Cortef |
| prednisone | Deltasone |
| triamcinolone | Aristocort |
| cortisone (naturally occurring) | Cortate |
| hydrocortisone | Cortef |

*Cyprohedptadines (allergy relief)*

| *Generic name:* | *Brand name:* |
|---|---|
| cyproheptadine HCl | Periactin |

*Anti-diabetic agents*

| *Generic name:* | *Brand name:* |
|---|---|
| (a) Insulin | Actrapid |
| | Humulin |
| | Velosulin |
| | Promatime |
| | Ultralente |
| (b) Sulfonylureas | |
| chlorpropamide | Diabinese |
| glipizide | Minidiab |
| tolbutamide | Rastinon |

*Phenothiazenes (anti-psychotics)*

| *Generic name:* | | *Brand name:* |
|---|---|---|
| chlorpromazine | | Largactil |
| prochlorperazine | | Stemetil |

*Tricyclic anti-depressants*

| *Generic name:* | | *Brand name:* |
|---|---|---|
| amitriptyline | | Endep |
| | | Tryptanol |
| clomipramine | | Anafranil |
| dothiepin | | Prothiaden |
| imipramine | | Tofranil |

*Oral contraceptives\**

| *Type of pill (oestrogen content):* | | *Brand name:* |
|---|---|---|
| Combined | (30µg and under) | Microgynon 30 |
| | (35µg) | Brevnor |
| | | Modicon |
| | | Nordette |
| | (50µg) | Microgynon 50 |
| | | Neogynon |
| | | Orthor Novum |
| | | Ovulen |
| Phased | (30–50µg) | Biphasil |
| | | Synphasic |
| | | Triquilar |

*Hormone replacement therapy (HRT) medications\**

| *Generic name:* | *Brand name:* |
|---|---|
| (a) Oestrogen | |
| conjugated oestrogens | Premarin |
| ethinyloestradiol | Estigyn |
| | Primogyn C |
| oestradiol | Oestradiol implants |
| (b) Progesterone | |
| levonorgestrel | Microlut |
| | Microval |
| medroxyprogesterone | Depo-Provera |
| norethisterone | Micronor |
| | Primalut |

*Note:* * Certain of these medications may cause fat gain in some women only.

in about 40 per cent of cases, but because these people have lost a lot more initially, the absolute regain is even greater.

Dr Judith Stern and her colleagues from New York University have tested the differences between a large group of women who have not deviated in weight by more than 3.6kg over several years on a fat loss program, and those who were 'regainers', i.e. who lost and regained at least 20 per cent of their weight within the same time period. They also looked at animal research to get some physiological indication of the reasons for the differences.[22]

The most striking difference the researchers found between regainers and maintainers was the use of exercise by the latter.

Around 76 per cent of those who were successful at keeping weight off over the long term had built exercise into their lifestyle compared with only 36 per cent of those who had failed. More maintainers than regainers (73–40 per cent) had also developed a personal eating plan as a lifestyle habit, whereas more regainers had used structured 'diet' programs, followed prescription from doctors, or used advice from books or magazines. Regainers snacked more during the day, and used chocolate and candy more often as their usual snack.

The other major difference between these groups and a control group of women who had never had a weight problem was in psychological techniques of coping with stress. The controls and those who were able to maintain their weight usually dealt with difficult situations by problem solving or confronting the issue. Significantly more regainers on the other hand used escape/avoidance techniques such as sleeping, eating or not dealing with the problem, in response to stress. This is consistent with other research that suggests that unless adequate coping skills are developed, individuals who don't make behaviour changes will return to their former negative pattern when a high-risk situation develops.[23]

These three factors: lifestyle changes in eating patterns, regular exercise and successful coping techniques are now recognised as key factors for long term maintenance of fat loss. In addition, Stern and her colleagues have shown that weight cycling through 'yo-yo' dieting and 'exercise cycling' (i.e. exercising for a period and then stopping) may have long term effects on dietary fat preference and fat intake. These are, therefore, also long term dangers for maintenance and re-inforce the fact that long term techniques of fat loss, to be successful, must incorporate long term changes in lifestyle rather than short term aberrations such as dieting or exercise 'programs'.

Dr Tim Wadden, a psychologist from the University of Pennsylvania, has also analysed relapse and maintenance by studying the habits of those who are successful with fat loss over the long term.[24] He suggests that:

- although diet may be important in helping to lose weight, those who develop a lifetime pattern of exercise manage to keep it off better
- greater maintenance occurs in women who do long, regular (although not necessarily vigorous) exercise like walking
- people who regularly eat just one fatty food have no increased

risk of regaining. But those who eat two, might just as well eat six—all are a recipe for relapse.
- most successful weight loss maintainers:
  - — don't count calories, but develop a personal eating plan
  - — exercise regularly
  - — closely monitor their weight
  - — monitor their food intake
- Best maintenance comes from setting realistic goals. In some severely obese people, there may be biological limits to big reductions. Satisfaction with more modest goals can improve the situation.

## IMPLICATIONS

1. Ensure that physical activity (i.e. play) is maintained at a sufficient level during early adolescence to prevent fat cell hyperplasia.
2. Recognise the types and importance of critical stages in fat gain in individuals and possible means of preventing this.
3. Recognise the various stages in life at which critical periods for fat gain can occur and be prepared to act on these.
4. Encourage breast-feeding for nursing mothers.
5. Encourage appropriate activity and eating patterns during pregnancy and the immediate post partum period.
6. Learn to recognise up-coming periods that are likely to be highly stressful and develop stress reduction techniques for coping with these.
7. Develop modified physical activity programs for women moving into the post-menopausal stage along the lines of those characteristically used for men.
8. Provide compensatory activities for individuals who significantly reduce their involvement in organised sport.
9. Encourage more physical activity and decreased fat intake in middle-aged men.
10. Try to maintain body fat levels during festive periods and work on fat reduction after these periods have passed.
11. Seek professional help or deal with issues arising from bereavement or separation before attempting to deal with body fat levels.
12. Check medications and any contra-indications with fat loss, and if necessary, consult with a patient's medical practitioner to see if alternative medications are available.
13. Where medication which affects fat loss is necessary, it is

important to be aware that fat loss may therefore be more difficult despite positive changes in eating and exercise habits.

14. Suggest that clients discuss with their doctor the implications of prescribed drugs on fat loss.

15. Plateaus in fat loss should be recognised as inevitable but not necessarily permanent forms of physiological adaptation.

16. Clients should be taught to be encouraged by a *lack of fat gain* during plateauing periods, in contrast to a *continuing loss.*

17. Prescription for breaking through plateaus may include change of exercise or eating patterns in order to overcome physiological adaptations.

18. There needs to be increased awareness of the consequences of periods of disillusionment, particularly where these correspond with plateaus in fat loss.

# 19
# Drugs and surgical treatment

SUMMARY OF MAIN POINTS

- Drug and surgical treatments are often necessary in people with intractable obesity problems.

- Selection of patients for drug and surgical treatment is critical.

- Stimulant drugs and others sold 'over-the-counter' are generally ineffective for long term weight loss and are potentially dangerous.

- The most successful drug currently used for treating obesity is dex fenfluramine (Adifax).

- Surgical treatments of obesity can be divided into (a) those restricting gastric capacity or absorption, and (b) those cosmetically removing fat.

- One of the most successful recent surgical techniques, because of its simplicity and adjustability, is laproscopic banding of the stomach.

The main techniques used for the treatment of obesity and overfatness discussed to this point are nutritional management, physical activity and behaviour management. In some cases, however, these are insufficient alone and pharmaceutical or surgical treatments may be required. In general, these are reserved for severe and intractable cases where the probability of other methods being successful is low and where the consequences of obesity are great. Both approaches require specialist medical diagnosis and care, but it is important for anyone working in the general field of fat loss counselling to understand the options available and their advantages and limitations. This chapter presents a summary of pharmaceutical and surgical techniques. Specific references in each area are recommended for further information.[1,2]

## DRUG TREATMENTS

Slimming drugs date back to the nineteenth century. It was then that ephedrine, extracted from the Chinese plant *Ephedra Sinica* and taken in tea as a stimulant, was first reportedly used. Further experimentation with this led to the development of amphetamines, and in the 1930s it was noted that these had an appetite suppressant effect by acting on the appetite centre of the brain. Unfortunately, the amphetamine-based drugs were also discovered to have marked effects on the central nervous system and euphoric qualities with much potential for abuse and so their use is now narrowly restricted by legislation in most countries.

Since then, there has been a vast array of research aimed at drug treatments, all with an obvious view to the huge marketing potential of a 'magic' product. The drugs researched can be broadly classified into three categories:

1. The appetite suppressant drugs, which broadly fall into those that act on central catecholamine neurotransmitter systems within the brain and those that act on the serotonergic system
2. Drugs aimed at increasing energy expenditure
3. Drugs used for changing fat and carbohydrate metabolism.

### Selection of patients for drug treatment

Drug treatment for obesity falls into a philosophical 'no-man's land' when it comes to patient selection. On the one hand, it has been argued that obesity should be like any other lifestyle risk factor such as hypertension and high blood cholesterol and treated with drugs automatically if lifestyle measures fail. Blood pressure and cholesterol are just like body fat, the argument goes, because excess levels of all of them are mainly due to the interaction between a susceptible genotype and a 'pathological' environment and they all have serious health consequences. Drs Ravussin and Bogardus from Phoenix, Arizona, have highlighted the similarity with essential hypertension (with no apparent secondary cause) by labelling some obesity as 'essential' obesity.[3] Protagonists in this argument say that obese people are discriminated against because obesity carries connotations of sloth and gluttony and all that is needed is a bit of self-help.

On the other hand, governments and medical insurance companies are very reluctant to pay for drug treatment of obesity. A simple calculation of the number of obese and overweight people multiplied by the cost of the drug sends them ducking for cover or bouncing the question back and asking which drugs should come off the subsidised list to allow the obesity drugs on and still remain within the budget. Needless to say, the full gamut of options between the two extremes are used to select patients for drug treatment.

One lesson which is slowly being taken from blood pressure and cholesterol drug treatment to obesity treatment is the concept of absolute risk. The question doctors are asking more and more before prescribing drugs is not 'how high is the person's blood pressure or cholesterol?', but 'at this level of blood pressure or cholesterol, what is the patient's risk of a heart attack or stroke?' To answer the first question, one only needs to measure the parameter being treated, but to answer the second question one needs to look at the patient and factor in the patient's age, sex, past history, smoking habits and the like. For blood pressure and cholesterol, there are tables available to insert all of these factors and come up with an overall assessment of cardiovascular risk to treat the blood pressure or cholesterol on that basis. Unfortunately, such tables are not available for obesity, but clearly, the assessment should include:

- body size, e.g. BMI
- fat distribution, e.g. WHR
- complications, e.g. diabetes, hypertension
- impact of obesity on physical, psychological and social functions
- other relevant factors such as family history of obesity and complications and personal history of weight gain and loss.

The overall extent of overfatness and its consequences can then be evaluated for each individual and this forms the basis for treatment decisions, especially those which can have significant negative as well as positive effects such as drug treatment and surgery.

## Types of drugs

### 1. Appetite suppressant drugs

This includes many 'over-the-counter' type weight loss products which often are stimulant based (using caffeine). Most are thus ineffective and potentially dangerous if taken over the long term. Where appetite is temporarily suppressed through stimulant action, this is generally compensated for by a decrease in metabolism and an increase in appetite on cessation of use. The addictiveness and tolerance effects of these drugs is also a potential problem.

Cholinergic neurotransmitter drugs include mazindol (Teronac, Sanorex), phentermine (Duromine, Ionamin) and phenylprop-anolamine. These have clear appetite suppressant activity and much less of a stimulant effect than amphetamines. Several trials have shown that they are effective in obese people over the short term in reducing subjective ratings of appetite, although like all such drugs, they must be combined with a low energy diet. Abuse appears to be low and there is a low incidence of side effects.

More recently, two other centrally acting drugs, fenfluramine and dex fenfluramine (brand name Adifax) have shown promise and have been widely researched. These are chemically related to the amphetamines but do not stimulate the central nervous system, so have less potential for abuse. They both increase seratonin transmission in the appetite centre by inhibiting its uptake into nerves—the way in which it is normally used. Seratonin then gives a feeling of satiety, so patients are still hungry, but are satisfied more easily.

The fenfluramines may be useful for small weight losses (i.e. around 0.2kg/week for the first few months), but only as long as the drug is taken. It needs to be withdrawn slowly, however, and may result in depression in some instances. It can be useful for

---

MYTH-INFORMATION

*Electric muscle stimulators are sometimes used in an attempt to duplicate the physical effort of muscles and therefore to burn fat. However, the electrical stimulus required at the skin level would need to be unbearably high to have this effect. These devices may also cause heart attacks and other medical complications in untrained hands.*

---

patients who are likely to be highly motivated and who would maintain any gains made from short term treatment with long term changes in lifestyle. This drug is currently regarded as perhaps the safest and most effective of the anti-obesity medications.[4]

Other possibilities in appetite control come from new work in a range of different areas,[5] and perhaps even through the recent discovery of the protein 'leptin' associated with the 'satiety gene' (see Chapter 16). However, the research unfolding from this original finding is making the future of this direction in drug research somewhat unclear.

## 2. Energy expenditure increasing drugs

Thyroid hormones were originally tried as a metabolism booster, but they caused a significant loss of lean mass and had frequent side effects. More recently, beta adrenergic agonists, designed to speed up the rate of fat lipolysis have shown promise for speeding up metabolism and these have attracted much popular media attention. The first round of these types of drugs was unsuccessful, largely because much of the weight lost was lean rather than fat tissue. Also they had a wide range of side effects such as tremor. A major concern is that if they are successful in increasing metabolism, this would lead to an excessive decrease in muscle, which in turn would lead to a decrease in metabolism, thus in the long run leading to more fat and less muscle. More research currently needs to be carried out in this area.

## 3. Drugs for changing fat and carbohydrate metabolism

These include the bulking agents to give a feeling of fullness (such as fibre tablets, many of which are now banned), and drugs aimed at changing the action of enzymes involved in the laying down and breaking up of fat in the fat cells. So far these have had only limited success, with perhaps the enzyme inhibitors (e.g. Acarbose) being the most successful. A new drug, tetrahydrolipostatin (HTL) currently being tested works by blocking the conversion of triglycerides to fatty acids. Without this step, fat can't be digested and hence not all the energy is taken in with the fat. These drugs, in theory, allow obese people to satisfy their taste for high-energy fatty foods, without absorbing all the calories. Concerns are already being raised, however, about the impact the extra fat will have on the large intestine and on the colonic bacteria involved in digestion. An imbalance of the colonic flora could mean an increase in the risk of abnormalities such as bowel cancer.

## SURGICAL TREATMENTS

Surgery is an option in motivated patients who are morbidly obese (those whose weight is 80 per cent or 45kg above ideal body weight) and in whom conservative treatments such as dieting have failed or those who have medical problems such as diabetes, high blood pressure or bad backs which might be substantially improved by massive weight reduction. The surgeon has only three methods of producing weight loss available to him. These methods are:

1. By restricting gastric capacity and so reducing the amount of food that a person can eat—the so-called gastric partitioning procedures.
2. By changing the intestinal tract so that food ingested is not properly digested or absorbed and so is lost from the body— the malabsorptive procedures.
3. By surgically removing areas of fat by excising them (lipectomy) or sucking out the fat (liposuction). This is classified as cosmetic rather than weight reducing.

### 1. Partitioning procedures or gastroplasties

These produce a small stomach pouch of 15–30cc connected to the lower part of the stomach by a narrow opening or 'stoma'. The effect of these procedures is to limit the patient to a very small meal which empties only slowly through the narrow stoma producing a feeling of satiety lasting 3–4 hours. Total daily food intake is, therefore, vastly reduced.

In order to achieve a good weight reduction with these procedures, patients must be prepared to make sacrifices and to be disciplined in the way in which they eat. This is not an easy way out and the patient must be strongly motivated to lose weight otherwise they may not feel that the sacrifices are worth while. They must:

- Adhere to a diet of easily masticated foodstuffs such as cereals, vegetables and white meats. Red meat is difficult to eat and the diet can seem boring.
- Measure food volumes and eat no more than 5 dessertspoons of food per meal. To eat more may cause vomiting and may stretch the pouch.
- Chew each small mouthful of food to a pulp before swallowing

otherwise the food pieces may block the stoma causing vomiting and pain.

- Avoid high calorie semi-liquid foods such as chocolate and ice cream as these liquefy and pass rapidly through the stoma, causing weight regain or preventing weight loss.
- Avoid solids when rushed or upset as vomiting is more likely in this situation.
- Take daily multivitamins and occasionally take iron if required.

With discipline, excellent weight reduction can be achieved with the average loss being 35kg and some patients losing much more. Two common methods used are 'stapling' and 'banding'.

### Gastric stapling

With stapling, the pouch is produced by placing a line of staples down the upper part of the stomach from just below the point where the gullet joins it and placing a piece of nylon mesh or tubing around, opening at the lower end. This stops the opening (stoma) enlarging. In many cases this type of procedure has produced satisfactory weight loss. However, it is a complex and difficult procedure. In the postoperative phase, complications such as leakage from the staple line and abscess formation may occur. Later the staple line may break down or the mesh erode into the stomach allowing food to pass through as normal, since restriction is lost. The result is often that lost weight is regained. Other complications include excessive vomiting and acid reflux causing heartburn. These are often caused by the pouch stretching. The operation is difficult to reverse when complications occur, as the staples can only be bypassed and not fully removed.

### Gastric banding or band gastroplasty

Gastric banding was developed to try to simplify the procedure. Instead of inserting a row of staples to create a pouch, a synthetic band is drawn around the upper stomach narrowing it at a point about 3cm below the junction of the gullet and stomach. This creates a small pouch with a narrow stoma just as with gastric stapling. There is less chance of stomach perforation, no staple line to break down and the procedure can be readily reversed by removing the band. Other problems such as erosion, excessive vomiting, pouch enlargement and reflux can still occur.

This procedure has now been further improved by the introduction of the laparascopically insertable (i.e. key hole surgery) adjustable silastic gastroplasty band (lap band). The band is clipped

**Figure 19.1: Gastric stapling**

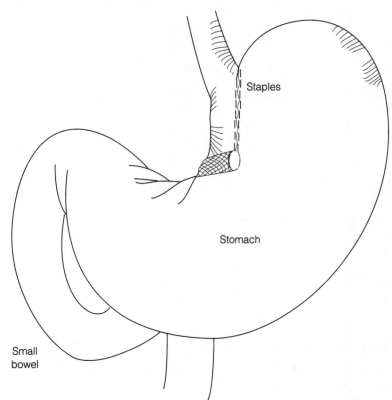

*Source:* Kraal (1989)[2]

around the upper stomach. It has a fixed circumference of about 10cm. The size of the stoma is adjusted by means of a circular balloon running around the inner surface of the band. This is connected via a fine tube to a reservoir (injection port) which is implanted in the abdominal wall muscle. Injection of saline fluid into or removal of fluid from the port tightens or opens the stoma. This adjusts the rate at which the pouch empties and allows fine tuning of the operation. It is the only laparascopically insertable and adjustable procedure available at present.

Unfortunately, either because of lack of patient motivation or compliance or because of technical problems, gastric partitioning procedures do have a failure rate of about 25 per cent requiring revision, reversal or conversion to another procedure. In these cases a malabsorptive procedure called biliopancreatic diversion is often recommended.

**Figure 19.2: Diagrammatic representation of the lap band**

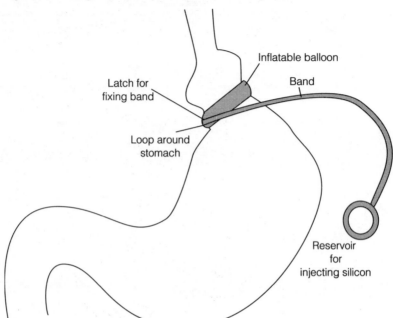

## 2. Biliopancreatic diversion

Biliopancreatric diversion has a number of elements:

- Part of the stomach is removed leaving a pouch of between 200–400cc. This reduces the volume of food that can be eaten but not as drastically as with gastric partitioning.
- The small bowel is divided at a point 250cm from where it enters the large bowel. This lower part of the small bowel is attached to the stomach pouch so that food from the stomach has a shorter length of small bowel to digest it before it enters the colon.
- The upper 3–4 metres of small bowel is attached to the lower large bowel at a point 50cm from where it joins the colon. This part of the bowel carries the digestive juices from the liver and pancreas. Instead of having the usual 5–6 metres of small bowel to mix with and digest the food, the digestive juices can only act on the food for a distance of 50cm.
- The gallbladder, if present, is removed.

The effect of these measures is to produce restriction of food intake and to cause malabsorption of the food that is eaten,

**Figure 19.3: Bileopancreatic diversion**

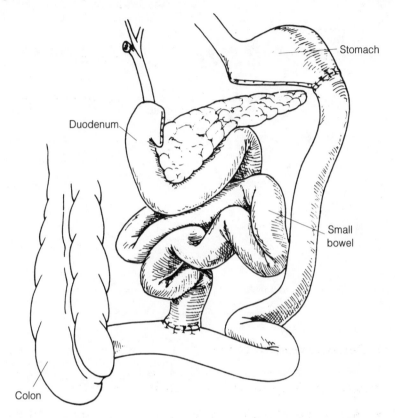

*Source:* Kraal (1989)[2]

particularly of fats. Initially the effect is rapid weight reduction often accompanied by diarrhoea and feelings of weakness. However, by twelve months, the body adjusts allowing normal sized meals of any food types to be eaten and bowel actions to stabilise at about three bowel actions per day. Often adult onset diabetes and high cholesterol are cured by this procedure. There is no problem with acid reflux or vomiting. Weight control is well maintained even ten years after surgery. However, it is a major operation with risk of leaks, abscesses, adhesions, etc, in the short term, and of deficiencies of protein, iron, calcium and vitamins long term. Patients must remain under review and have six-monthly blood tests so that any developing deficiencies may be detected early and supplements prescribed to correct the problem before it becomes serious.

**Table 19.1: A summary of fat surgery pros and cons**

| Type | Explanation | Advantages | Disadvantages |
|---|---|---|---|
| **A. Food limiting** | | | |
| Gastric stapling | Produces a small pouch joined to lower stomach by narrow, slow draining opening restricting food volume | Simple concept. Food passes into lower stomach as normal and lower pouch may be checked | Risk of leakage, staple line may breakdown, may develop reflux and excess vomiting. Difficult to reverse, needs motivation |
| Fixed sized banding | As above | As above plus inexpensive and less invasive than stapling. Easy to reverse | May develop reflux and vomiting. Erosion of band. Needs motivation. Restriction of food varieties. Not adjustable |
| Lap band | As above | Adjustable and inserted by laprascope. Rapid recovery and minimal pain | As above, although erosion less likely. May slip in early post-op. period |
| Biliopancreatic bypass | Produces restriction of food volume and malabsorption of food eaten, especially fats | Better sustained weight loss with less vomiting and potential cure of reflux, diabetes and high cholesterol. Can eat normal food in normal sized helpings after 1 year | More major surgery with risk of more complications. Loose bowel actions. Loss of nutrients requiring lifelong supervision and supplements |
| **B. Surgical removal** | | | |
| Lipectomy (arm, thigh, breast, abdomen | Fat cut-off surgically | Moderate amounts reduced quickly | Fat can return in other places; scarring; may be left with layers of skin |
| Liposuction | Fat 'sucked out' | Limited scarring; can remove unsightly pockets | Bruising; uneven removal in some cases; only small amounts can be taken at a time; possible return of fat cell growth |

## 3. Techniques aimed at surgically removing fat

These are known best as the 'plastic surgery' techniques. They involve removing fat by (a) cutting it off (called 'lipectomy') or (b) 'sucking' it out (called 'liposuction'). These techniques have typically been used on females, but up to 25 per cent of patients are now male, particularly looking for abdominal fat reductions.

## Lipectomy

Fat is removed from under the skin through a surgical incision, and the skin pulled tighter over the area. The process is used on the thighs, arms, abdomen and breasts and up to 5kg of fat can be removed at a time. There is a concern though that fat may return to other parts of the body and that post-operative care must be paid to diet and exercise.

## Liposuction

Liposuction involves 'sucking' fat cells from a small incision with a vacuum-like apparatus. Only small amounts can be taken at a time (e.g. up to 1kg) and for this reason it is used as a 'body sculpting' procedure rather than a significant fat loss operation. Liposuction causes bruising and can leave an uneven result in the hands of less skilled surgeons, although scarring from cutting is less.

There have been a number of other surgical techniques used to deal with obesity over the years, many in an experimental attempt to find an appropriate procedure. By 1993 there were 43 different operational procedures or modifications used in such a way. Recently, criteria have been established for accepting such procedures, and these have resulted in a number now being regarded as of questionable value including the following:

> . . . tooth wiring, acupuncture, hypothalamic centre manipulation, liposuction, balloon insertion, unbanded gastric partitioning, vagotomy, gastrogastrostomy, horizontal gastroplasty, gastric wrap, gastroclip and any variety of gastroplasty without a reinforced stoma, intestinal bypass, duodenal bypass and biliointestinal bypass.[6]

Surgical treatment of obesity is therefore limited, but some procedures may be of use in intractable cases of obesity in combination with other standard fat loss procedures.

## IMPLICATIONS

1. Pharmaceutical approaches to fat loss should be seen as having potential value only when other conventional fat loss techniques have failed.
2. Pharmaceutical and surgical techniques must be accompanied by an eating and physical activity plan.
3. Diagnosis and long term maintenance of pharmaceutical and

surgical techniques must be carried out under the care of the appropriate professionals.

4. Pharmaceutical approaches are currently only used for short term treatment and patient selection is important.

5. All over-the-counter medications for fat loss should be avoided, particularly for extended use.

6. Stimulant drugs for fat loss have the potential for addiction and tolerance formation and therefore should be avoided.

7. Topical applications with claims for fat loss must comply with the appropriate regulations under the poisons act.

8. Any use of surgery for obesity must be accompanied by the appropriate medical advice.

9. Neither pharmaceutical nor surgical treatments should be seen as a panacea for fat loss and should only be entered into after a full evaluation of benefits and risks.

# 20

# Eating disorders

## SUMMARY OF MAIN POINTS

- Obsession with dieting and weight control can lead to eating disorders.
- There is no evidence that educational efforts to reduce obesity increase eating disorders in a community.
- The main eating disorders are anorexia nervosa and bulimia.
- These exist in about 1–10 per cent of the female population. Anorexia and bulimia are currently not common in males though they certainly occur.
- Disordered eating patterns for bulking, as in body building, are more characteristic of males.
- Eating disorders as a side effect must be considered in any fat loss programming.

Any discussion of weight control or fat loss programs would not be complete without a consideration of eating disorders. These may be an inevitable consequence of the idea that we can sculpt our bodies and 'will' our minds to accomplish any ideal without any apparent downside. The move towards a 'perfect' body is exacerbated by images portrayed in the media and by careers or professions, such as gymnastics and dancing, where an extremely slim or lean physique is required. However, whilst an unrealistic body ideal is a trigger for eating disorders, there is no evidence that initiatives to reduce obesity in the community *per se*, have this effect. Eating disorders have been reported in the literature for hundreds of years, well before the time of the modern obsession with weight.

The two main disorders to be considered here are *anorexia nervosa*, and *bulimia*. Because these are specialty areas of study, the discussion here is necessarily brief and directed towards the practical implications for fat loss leaders working with clients who may manifest these problems. Readers are referred to more specialist texts or journals for a more detailed analysis of eating disorders.[1,2]

## ANOREXIA NERVOSA AND BULIMIA

Anorexia nervosa is essentially an *under*-eating disorder in contrast to the *over*-eating problems associated with the development of obesity. Bulimia is essentially a *mal*-eating disorder, as is the obsessive over-eating of specific nutrients that is associated with bulking, such as in body building, which will not be discussed in detail here.[3,4] This latter pattern of mal-eating is more likely to occur in males because of the social ideal of bulk in men. The vast majority (90 per cent) of sufferers from anorexia and bulimia are women, although it is acknowledged that this may change in the future with changes in social and gender attitudes.

Both anorexia and bulimia have potentially severe, and possibly fatal consequences. Amongst individuals admitted to hospital for anorexia, the mortality is more than 10 per cent, death resulting usually from starvation, suicide or electrolyte imbalance. The long term outcome of bulimia is unknown, but disturbed eating behaviour may last for several years. Both anorexia and bulimia focus the individual's attention almost exclusively on dissatisfaction with one's own body size and shape, idealising the thin, androgynous figure and equating this with success, happiness, strength and discipline, and fat with failure and lack of attractiveness. The inter-relationship between anorexia and bulimia is complex. Some anorexia sufferers will at times binge and vomit and some bulimia sufferers have also suffered from anorexia, although they may now be normal weight.

For the counsellor, there may be times of concern as to what constitutes a 'healthy' attitude towards body maintenance, fat loss and eating, as opposed to a dysfunctional one. Both anorexic and bulimic clients may present themselves for assistance with weight loss, body building and exercise programs, any of which may inadvertently feed their disorder.

---

**MYTH-INFORMATION**

*Massage can help improve circulation and enhance relaxation, however it has no long term physical effect on body fat loss or fitness.*

---

## Anorexia nervosa

*Anorexia nervosa* is defined as a condition of under-nutrition predisposing to extreme thinness. The prevalence of anorexia and bulimia in the general community is relatively low with between 1–10 per cent of females ever being classified as suffering from the disorder.[5] These figures though may hide the higher level of dietary obsessions which occur without manifesting as a genuine eating disorder. As up to 40 per cent of females and 24 per cent of males admit to currently dieting to lose weight,[6] it could be assumed that many of these may be abnormally restricting food input. On the other hand, the abundance of high energy foods in modern Western societies implies that at least some dietary restraint must be undertaken by almost everybody at some point and hence restrained eating cannot be defined as an eating disorder *per se*. Pathologically predisposing forms of restrained eating are defined by a number of psychological tests and diagnostic criteria.

### *Diagnostic criteria*[7]

The following symptoms are considered to be characteristic of anorexia:

- a relentless pursuit of thinness
- a significant degree of weight loss (up to 15 per cent below average) weight for height
- an intense fear of becoming obese
- disturbance of body image ('feels' fat even when emaciated)
- a refusal to maintain body weight over a minimal normal for age and height
- no known physical illness that would account for weight loss
- usually amenorrhea in women and diminished sexual activity in men.

The are two main types of anorexia: (a) the 'restricting' type in which the individual does not regularly engage in bingeing or purging behaviour and (b) the binge-eating/purging type in which the individual regularly engages in bingeing or purging, self-induced vomiting or misuse of laxatives, diuretics or enemas. In addition, the International Classification of Health Disorders has recently defined a third type, characterised by no major restriction of food input, but by excessive exercise. This has been labelled 'exercise anorexia'.

In anorexia, the client rarely presents as having a problem being too thin. The denial of the diagnosis of anorexia is usually accompanied by a sense of mastery over the body and its attempts to restore equilibrium through eating. There is often a kind of 'magical' thinking in which the sufferer thinks she is free from the normal requirements of food and drink, and can continue to starve herself without any ill effects. The complex causes of anorexia, which may include family dysfunction, personality disturbances, a perception of self as 'helpless' or 'powerless', as well as dissatisfaction with size and shape, is further complicated and maintained by the effects of starvation itself.

### Bulimia

The desire to maintain a sub-optimal weight also frequently underlies the condition of bulimia, although bulimia sufferers are usually close to normal weight for height. Bulimia is defined as a behaviour involving a variety of techniques for purging after binge-eating. Unlike those who suffer from obesity or anorexia with associated body size, there are few clues to the condition of bulimia for the observer. For this reason its prevalence is probably much higher than estimated, and its diagnosis is more difficult. Its prevalence (1–3 per cent amongst adolescent and young females) is thought to have significantly increased during the last 20 years, with surveys in the US indicating possibly as many as 15 per cent of college aged women experiencing some form of bulimia.[8] Many bulimia sufferers seek treatment only after years of binge-eating and vomiting, feeling both responsible for and guilty and ashamed of their disorder. On the other hand, clients may seek help for weight loss without ever disclosing the underlying condition.

*Diagnostic criteria*

The following symptoms are considered to be characteristic of bulimia:

- usually normal weight-for-height—but may be slightly over or under weight
- morbid fear of fatness
- extreme sensitivity to weight gain
- recurrent episodes of bingeing (characterised by the feeling of loss of control over eating) followed by self-induced vomiting—at least twice a week for three months
- purgative abuse—may be in addition to vomiting
- excessive exercise or fasting
- depressive symptoms.

Non-purging type bulimia may also occur, involving bingeing together with inappropriate compensatory behaviours such as fasting or excessive exercise, but not vomiting or laxative abuse. Possible medical complications of bulimia include dehydration, electrolyte abnormalities, salivary gland swelling, possible kidney disease, gastrointestinal problems, possible endocrine abnormalities, dental caries and erosion of tooth enamel.

## RECOGNISING EATING DISORDERS

The relationship between developing an eating disorder and 'dieting' is unclear, but it is generally accepted that both anorexia and bulimia tend to be preceded by a period of intense dieting, or food restriction. How or why this happens is uncertain, however, in laboratory conditions it can be demonstrated that 'dieters' will eat more than 'non-dieters' after they have consumed food which they believe to be low in calories. This process, known as 'counter-regulation', seems to suggest that there is a strong cognitive component in the maintenance of these disorders. In both anorexia and bulimia, the sufferer eats according to extreme dietary restrictions. Anything which interferes with these self-imposed rules (believing they have eaten something 'wrong', depression, anxiety or stress) results in a temporary total abandonment of control. The type of foods chosen at these times (the 'forbidden' foods) not only alleviate distress, but may also provide significant pleasure, a factor which reinforces both their use as a binge food and their banishment from the path of 'true dieting'. Subsequent to the binge, seen as proof that the body and its appetites cannot be trusted, there is an even more fervent return to rigidly controlled dieting.

Both bulimia and anorexia are complex in their aetiology and resistant to treatment. It seems likely that there is no one underlying cause and that psychological, physiological and social factors are involved in both the development and maintenance of the disorders. It is seen as significant that both conditions are primarily female disorders, linked to the psychological, social and cultural emphasis given to how a woman looks, as opposed to how she feels. Female (role) models continue to present young women with body sizes and shapes which are unachievable by the majority. The problem is probably also intergenerational as research shows that many young women identify with their own mothers' pre-occupation with their bodies and their mothers may project their body image concerns onto their daughters.[9]

By the age of 18 it is estimated that 80 per cent of females have started dieting. Many of these women have discovered bulimia themselves even without being shown or told by peers or the media. Few have any idea of the potential consequences of their attempts to fix their weights at sub-optimal levels. For these women, dieting takes the place of dealing with more serious issues such as their self-esteem and body image disturbance, the transition to adult sexuality, the development of an autonomous self and the initiation of intimate relationships, dysfunctional family sequelae, mood disturbances and ongoing stress management. More recently, it has been suggested that a high proportion of women with eating disorders have a background of sexual and/or physical abuse.[10]

## ISSUES FOR THE FAT LOSS COUNSELLOR

There is no way at present to distinguish between individuals who will or will not develop an eating disorder subsequent to dieting. There is also no way to identify who will or will not be damaged by repeated weight cycling. It is uncertain whether some people will need constant support and monitoring to maintain fat loss. It may be that a different approach needs to be taken for people with a food dependence from the traditional approaches used in behavioural and self-management practice.

A further model for eating disorders has been proposed with reference to obesity and non-purging bulimia, which suggests that repeated cycles of dieting and regaining weight lead to food dependence.[11] Dependence is defined as 'the failure to stop using a substance that is deleterious to health and where use results in short term mood alteration'. In this model, food (specifically those foods which are reserved for bingeing episodes) becomes a psychoactive substance. In common with other psychoactive addictions it has the following characteristics:

- food is used in larger amounts, or for longer periods than the person intended
- there is a persistent desire or effort to cut down or control intakes
- there is a continued use of a food despite the knowledge that there is a persistent or recurrent physical, social or psychological problem caused by its consumption
- there are 'withdrawal' symptoms—cravings, anxiety, tension, depression—when the food is not available

Obese and bulimic clients frequently report bingeing in response to stress, frustration, rejection or other negative emotional states, and it seems likely that both uncontrolled eating and the kinds of food used (high carbohydrate/fat) act synergistically to lower the internal arousal state. Few of these clients are able to activate behavioural self-management techniques at these times.

This presents the fat loss counsellor with a major dilemma; on the one hand is the desire to encourage healthy weight loss, but on the other is the concern about encouraging restrictive eating disorders. Unless the counsellor turns away a client, leaving them at the mercy of someone less scrupulous, they have a responsibility to be helpful, and above all, to do no harm. The following are some guidelines for counsellors, based on this 'do-no-harm' principle:

## MYTH-INFORMATION

*Tai Chi, the ancient Chinese art of movement, is a form of relaxation which may, indirectly, have an effect on nervous eating and thereby improve body fat levels. The physical component of Tai Chi alone, however, is not sufficient to create a significant energy deficit.*

## GUIDELINES

1. Develop and maintain good rapport and listening skills.
2. Clearly define the services you or your organisation offer, i.e. no 'quick fixes', magic formulae or 'diets'.
3. When taking a client's history, always ask about prior expe-

riences of dieting, bulimia or anorexia. Identify present behaviours associated with eating, emotional triggers for over-eating or bingeing, and whether bulimia is practised currently. The following questions may be useful:

- Have you ever suffered from an eating disorder?
- Has any member of your family had an eating disorder?
- Do you ever binge eat? Do you ever make yourself sick afterwards?
- If yes, what sort of things trigger you to do this?

4. Always refer on someone about whom you have concerns for psychological/psychiatric assessment. Be prepared to work in a supportive role if therapy is necessary.
5. Explore with a client their expectations of dieting and fat loss. Be particularly attentive to unrealistic expectations such as, the speed with which they imagine it will happen, and how they will feel if fat loss does not occur.
6. Your client is entitled to make an informed choice about his or her treatment; you need to explain the current low success rates for long term behavioural maintenance of fat loss (i.e. 5–25 per cent) and the difference between working on this as opposed to long term lifestyle changes, which may not reduce their fat significantly, but may improve well-being.
7. Do not encourage or focus on dieting. If a client is severely obese, he or she will probably need medical assistance to deal with the problem, and referral to the appropriate service is called for. For most clients, however, the most important help you can give is to gently challenge their 'diet' mentality.
8. Be prepared to counter resistance with 6!
9. Before beginning any change or process have a client keep a record of what they are eating now. Focus on problem times and meals.
10. Institute changes one at a time.

## DEALING WITH AN EATING DISORDER.

If an eating disorder is suspected in a client a counsellor should:

1. CHECK your perception with a colleague. Describe the behaviour that makes you concerned, without identifying the person, as a hypothetical case. Find out if they would have the same concern.
2. MAINTAIN rapport and relationship with the client.

3. IDENTIFY likely resources in the community to whom you could refer your client. Talk to the professional concerned, again to check your perception of the problem. Notify him or her that you may be referring someone.
4. CHOOSE a time to talk to the client in which you will not be pressured or disturbed and a place which is free from interruptions and is confidential. Notify the switchboard/receptionist that you won't be available for a little while.
5. LET your client know of your concern and ask if it is OK to discuss the problem. If your client accepts that it is a legitimate concern and is prepared to talk with you, continue to facilitate his or her exploration. Ask if they would be prepared to see another health professional to ascertain what, if any, is appropriate treatment. Keep the focus on developing a healthy sense of self and body, rather than on morbidity or illness. Give your client the professional's phone number and leave them with the task of making an appointment.

If the client denies there is a problem, especially if the suspected eating disorder is anorexia, ask if there is anyone else who they can talk to about it. Clearly outline the reasons for your concern (for instance, demonstrate where the client is placed on the healthy weight range) and your own disquiet about the situation. Suggest that maybe you could talk about it after they have had time to consider what you have said. Keep a rapport. Be prepared to be firm as well as gentle. This process may need to be repeated several times.

Gyms, fitness centres and lifestyle programs all need a policy of handling of suspected eating disorders so as to promote healthy, rather than inappropriate eating and exercise routines. This policy needs to include guidelines for referral, limitations on the use of exercise machines, weights etc. and the use of broadly based food choices as opposed to diets.

# 21

# Ethical issues in obesity treatment

SUMMARY OF MAIN POINTS

- Ethical issues need to be understood and carefully assessed by professionals dealing with fat loss.
- A common principle of ethical decision-making is 'do no harm'.
- Ethical considerations must include yourself, your client, the resources available and the social context.

Research revealing the side effects of dieting and the poor long term effectiveness of fat loss programs has altered the way we think about dealing with obesity as a health problem. We now know that fat loss programs carry some real risks and some authors have suggested that the treatment of obesity may be unethical.[1] Certainly the ethical issues need to be understood and carefully assessed by professionals dealing with fat loss.

## Is obesity treatment safe and effective?

High rates of fat loss are achievable in the short term but are rarely maintained. Consequently, many obese people find that their treatment creates fat fluctuations that may entrench their obesity.[2,3]

## Whose problem is obesity?

There is little doubt that obesity has many health consequences. Many overweight people, however, suffer few serious consequences that are a direct result of obesity. Obesity and its treatment are not simply issues of physical health; psychological and social issues must also be taken into account.

Many people who are unhappy with the shape of their bodies and want to lose fat have no obvious health problems associated with obesity. They may not even be significantly overweight. There are strong suggestions, particularly relevant to women, in advertising, entertainment, fashion and publishing that thinness is desirable and an indication of a successful life. Is it ethical for professionals to contribute to this pressure? Should we not instead be helping people to feel good about themselves irrespective of how they look, if the health risks seem minimal?

Pressure from others to lose fat raises ethical questions about individual freedom. Is it a right or a duty to be healthy? Should you be free to eat how and what you choose or do you have an obligation to society to eat healthily and meet normal criteria? Why should it be wrong for an obese person to enjoy a pleasure-giving chocolate bar, but right to follow someone's advice of going without, which would give a degree of displeasure?

## THE RESPONSIBILITIES OF PROVIDING ADVICE

When someone comes to you for help, they assume that you have the power to help them. How much power they provide you, as the professional, will depend on the individual. Some will expect you to be very powerful, perhaps able to bring about great changes and protect them from harm in the process. Others will expect less, seeing the power as being equally shared or confined to areas of knowledge and expertise that they believe themselves to lack. This may have little to do with your real powers but be an expression of the client's needs and habitual ways of dealing with other people. Of course, often you will have knowledge and expertise that the client lacks and they trust you to give advice that is safe, effective and appropriate.

You have an obligation to act responsibly with this power, especially where the client expects a lot or is unaware of how much they are putting themselves in your hands. You are often in the better position to understand any complications in managing his or her needs.

## ETHICS AND SUCCESSFULNESS

It is unlikely that there would be so much concern about the ethics of obesity treatment if the long term follow-up studies of fat loss programs were more optimistic about the sustainability of fat loss. It may not be honest to make general claims about the effectiveness of fat loss programs knowing that long term success may prove illusory.[4]

Judging success means establishing criteria for success. Who gets to choose these criteria is also an issue of power and there is little in the way of public consensus or professional standards of practice to protect clients or professionals. Your work with someone might result in her feeling much better about herself and improve her fitness, which you regard as a success, but she might complain that she failed to lose much fat, which was her criterion of success. Which of you is right? How would consumer protection legislation comment on this, were the dispute to go to court?

How you compare with your client on characteristics such as gender, race, intelligence, occupation, physical stature, wealth, and language affects whose point-of-view prevails in the selection of criteria for success. You might end up agreeing to a treatment that is ethically dubious because you are intimidated by a rich, beautiful or famous client. Alternatively, the client might be intimidated by you into accepting something she feels uncomfortable with. If neither you nor your client is aware that this might happen, there will be little you can do to protect yourselves from it.

## ETHICS, RISKS AND BENEFITS

A common guiding principle of ethical decision-making is to 'do no harm', Fat-reduction methods have a number of risks that should be balanced against the potential benefits for each client.[5,6]

For some people, for example those with diabetes or heart disease, the need to lose fat is paramount and the ethical balance is clearly in favour of attempting fat loss. Conversely, for some people the risks of losing fat, especially by dieting, are so great that the ethical balance is usually in favour of discouraging fat loss (for example, people with anorexia nervosa, binge-eating disorder or a history of cyclical dieting).

The decision will not be so obvious in most cases and you will need a good knowledge of the potential risks and benefits of your approach to fat loss methods as well as carrying out a careful assessment of each individual client.

## ETHICAL DECISION MAKING

The variability of people and the complexity of factors that cause a person to seek help with fatness means that there can be no standard set of rules. You have to make a fresh ethical decision with each new request for help, often even within the handling of one client. Frequently, these decisions need to be made on-the-spot, without the opportunity to seek advice.

It is important to have thought through a general framework for ethical decision-making in advance, that will assist with making on-the-spot judgements and decisions.

There are four domains which are important to consider:

- yourself
- the client
- the treatment resources available
- the social context.

You must also consider the interplay of these four domains.

### Yourself

Our past experiences and what we have made of them affect our reactions to people and situations. We see each new thing we encounter through a 'filter' of beliefs and expectations that helps us make sense of them. This in turn influences how we respond.

You need to know yourself well, especially your motives, attitudes and feelings regarding obesity, overeating, exercise and health. Failure to understand these things increases the risk that you will act unethically by unintentionally imposing your personal values on your clients.

What do you think is the most important outcome goal for this person? Why? In your work, you are pursuing your own goals as well as your clients'. This means that they hold some power over your job satisfaction—you cannot succeed without their active cooperation. This motivates you to shape their goals in line with your own objectives rather than being there simply for your client. If you are clearly aware of your own choice of goals in a particular case, you can more easily see any conflict between your own goals and those of your client.

What do you believe has made this client obese? How do you feel about that? Your theory about why a particular client is obese will play a big part in the actions you take. In reality, different people come to be obese along different paths, but the feelings that arise in you because of your theory are very important. For example, you might decide that a particular client is obese because during childhood she learned to select sweet and fatty foods in her diet, following her mother's choices. This theory may give you feelings that the client is 'not to blame' and that her mother was at fault. Indeed, you may have strong feelings about poor childhood nutrition and regard the mother as having been a poor parent or even somewhat abusive of the child for making her obese. This might lead to you feeling sorry for the client and trying to be the 'good parent' that her mother was not.

On the other hand, you might think that another client who has had good nutritional advice for years has remained obese because he has not put the advice into practice. This could give you feelings of hopelessness about working with him or even anger that he has wasted other busy helpers' time and is going to waste yours too.

Do you believe it would be possible to have the things that are important to you personally if you were as obese as this client? Usually, we think that the things that we personally value are desirable to others as well. If you believe that your client needs to lose fat in order to have a chance of getting something that you value in your life, you are less likely to consider or support alternative goals and means of achieving these. For example, the client might be concerned that she needs to lose fat in order to get a partner. If you believe that you would feel this way if you were equally obese, it may be difficult for you to work constructively with her feelings about personal attractiveness and relationships.

What skills do you have with which to respond to this client's needs? It is generally regarded as unethical to promise what one does not have the ability to provide. It is also your ethical responsibility to respond *appropriately* to a particular client's needs. It is possible, perhaps even quite common, for the client to have come to the wrong person for help—they are not always well-informed about their needs and the services that cater to these needs.

This question helps you to think about whether the client has realistic expectations of what you can do. The most ethical response to a particular client may be to decline her request for help and discuss more appropriate alternatives.

## The client

Your clients, like you, are human beings with complex motives and needs. Some of these will be well-understood by the clients and some will be more apparent to others than to themselves. It is not usually ethically acceptable to take clients at face value, especially when you are dealing with potentially very complex issues.

What is this client asking for? Why does he or she want that? With personal issues such as health, fitness and appearance the client's expression of his or her needs can easily be distorted by anxiety.

The woman in the above example who wishes to get a satisfying relationship by losing fat is unlikely to give this initially as her reason for seeking help. If she is partially aware of and embarrassed about her insecurities, she may deny this even if you ask directly about it. You need to take some care in considering what the initial request for help really represents.

What are his or her strengths and weaknesses? Consider what the client is and is not capable of achieving. Sometimes you can teach the skills and knowledge required. Sometimes the client already has these, so they can be left out of the program. Sometimes you can refer them to someone else who can offer better help or modify your approach accordingly.

What are the probable consequences of this client successfully losing fat? Of staying the same? You should consider whether the gains that can be reasonably expected would be a worthwhile return on the effort and cost involved. You should specifically take into account potential unwanted effects, particularly if the fat loss efforts are unsuccessful.[7] This should include some thought about how the client and other important people in her life are likely to respond to the client losing fat and how they would respond if she regained it. The responses will not always be entirely positive.

What is this client's history of obesity management? How have these past efforts affected them? Most clients have already made many efforts to lose fat. This history of efforts to lose fat makes up a powerful set of learning experiences that shape what clients expect of you and of themselves. Unless there is good reason to expect a different outcome, it may be unethical to repeat things that have been unhelpful in the past. It is almost certainly unethical to re-expose the client to something that has already been found to be harmful.

## The treatment resources available

Ethical decisions need to be realistic. That means they have to fit the actual circumstances rather than ideal circumstances. You need to take into account the actual treatment resources available, even if these differ from what would ideally be the case.

What treatment can you offer? This goes beyond consideration of your particular expertise and takes account of what you usually offer or any constraints imposed by the organisation for which you work.

What resources can you refer to? The ethics of offering help may differ according to the alternatives available. In circumstances where few other resources are available or your skills, however limited, exceed those of the available alternatives, it may be unethical not to offer help even though in the context of a richer range of alternatives, it would be ethical for you to refer on.[7]

## The social context

The significance of other people to both yourself and your client is an important source of information for your ethical decision-making. Everyone is motivated by the attitudes and opinions of others, especially those who are important in one's life.

How do the opinions and attitudes of others affect this client's goals? Obese clients often declare that they wish to lose fat because someone else wants them to, usually a partner but sometimes also another helper such as a physician. A careful examination of the relationship between the client and the other person will tell you something about the ethics of working with the client. For example, the extent to which the client wishes to lose fat for personal reasons, or feels forced into it, is likely to be relevant.

How do the opinions of others affect your goals? Everyone's job meets a variety of personal needs, including social ones. For example, a client may have been referred to you by someone you respect or value as a source of referrals and do not want to disappoint. You may feel the need to get a good result in order to secure your relationship with the referrer. This need to impress the referrer may make it difficult for you to turn the client down even if there are good reasons to do so. Conversely, you may feel the need to prove your effectiveness as a fat loss agent and may therefore avoid offering help to clients who appear unlikely to achieve impressive fat losses even though they could benefit greatly from your help in other ways.

## INFORMED CONSENT

The threat of the client's disempowerment in the helping process can be moderated by sharing the decision-making and risk-taking with the client. This is readily achieved through the process of informed consent.

The latin roots of consent, *con sentire*, mean 'to feel with'. Consent is about mutual understanding. You need to understand how the client sees his or her obesity and its causes, potential solutions, their self-image, skills, etc. You need to explain your own point of view on these issues, what skills you have to offer, and what treatment options are available and valid. Together, you and the client must negotiate a treatment plan that is the best amalgam of yourself, the client, the treatments, and the social context. The quality of the result of this negotiation is a major determinant of the ethics of the treatment.

## GAINING THE SKILLS TO ACT ETHICALLY

Ethical practice is achieved through a combination of attitudes and behaviour that can be learned through reading, discussion, reflection, training and practice. Meeting with colleagues to discuss work problems, particularly ethical anxieties, is a good way to compare your ethical thinking with others and develop confident approaches to practical issues. Training courses in communication and basic counselling skills are readily available. These can increase your understanding of the relationship between client and helper and will assist in the development of skills that promote ethical practice.

Regular application of the skills and concepts relevant to ethical practice, with periodic reflection on your development, will help ensure that this learning is consolidated.

# Notes

## 1 Overfatness and obesity into the 21st century

1 Bray, G., 1990, 'Epidemiology of obesity', In *Progress in Obesity Research*, John Libbey, London; Allied Dunbar, 1994, *National Fitness Survey*, Health Education Authority, HMSO, London.

2 National Heart Foundation of Australia, 1989, *Risk Factor Prevalence Study*, No 3, NHF, Canberra.

3 Stamler, J., 1993, 'Epidemic obesity in the United States', *Archives of Internal Medicine*, 153: 1040–1044.

4 Owen, N., Bauman A., 1992, 'The descriptive epidemiology of a sedentary lifestyle in adult Australians', *International Journal of Epidemiology*, 21: 305–310.

5 Hillary Commission, 1990, *Life in New Zealand Survey* (LINZ), Otago University.

6 Public Health Service, 1991, 'Promoting health/preventing disease' *Objectives for the nation*, US Govt Printing Office, Washington, DC.

7 Allied Dunbar, 1994, *National Health Service Survey*, UK Health Authority.

8 Hills, A., and Wahlqvist, M., 1994, 'What is overfatness', In Wahlqvist and Hills (eds), *Exercise and Obesity*, Smith-Gordon, London.

9 World Health Organisation, 1995, 'Physical status: The use and interpretation of anthropometry', *WHO Technical Report Series*, (in press).

10 Zimmett, P., Dowse, G., Serjeantson, S., King, H., 1990, 'The epidemiology and natural history of NIDDM—lessons from the South Pacific', *Diabetes/Metabolism Reviews*, 6:91–124.

11 Horm, J., Anderson, K., 1993, 'Who in America is trying to lose weight?', *Annals of Internal Medicine*, 119(7):672–676.

12 Williamson D.F. et al., 1992, 'Weight loss attempts in adults: Goals,

duration and rate of weight loss', *American Journal of Public Health*, 82:1251–1257.

13　Boyle, K., Dobson, A., Bennett, S., Egger, G., 1994, 'Can the increasing weight of Australians be explained by the decreasing prevalence of cigarette smoking?', *International Journal of Obesity*, 18:55–60.

14　Saris, W., 1995, 'Exercise and weight control', *Australian Society for the Study of Obesity, Annual Conference*, Melbourne.

15　Kuczmarski, R.J., Flegal, K.M., Campbell, S.M., & Johnson, C.L., 1994, 'Increasing prevalence of overweight among US adults: The National Health and Nutrition examination surveys, 1960 to 1991', *Journal of the American Medical Association* 272:205–211.

16　Bouchard, C., 1992, 'Etiology and pathogenesis: Genetic aspects of human obesities', In Belfiore, F., Jeanrenaud, B., Papalia, D. (eds), *Obesity: Basic concepts and clinical aspects*, Basel, Karger, 28–36.

## 2　Fat in health and disease

1　O'Dea, K., 1992, 'Obesity and Diabetes in the "Land of Milk and Honey" ', *Diabetes/Metabolism Reviews*, 8(4):373–388.

2　Colditz, G., 1992, 'The economic costs of obesity', *American Journal of Clinical Nutrition*, 55:5053–5075.

3　Vague, J., 1956, 'The degree of masculine differentiation of obesities: A factor determining predisposition of diabetes, atherosclerosis, gout and urine calculus disease', *American Journal of Clinical Nutrition*, 4:20.

4　Pi-Sunyer, F.X., 1993, 'Medical hazards of obesity', *Annals of Internal Medicine*, 119:655–660.

5　Rodin, J., 1992, 'Determinants of body fat localization and its implications for health', *Annals of Behavioural Medicine*, 14(4):275–281.

6　Allied Dunbar 1995, *National Survey*, 1995, Health Education Authority, London.

7　Editorial, 1991, 'The metabolic basis for the 'apple' and the 'pear' body habitus', *Nutrition reviews*, 49(3):84–86.

8　Despres, J-P et al., 1995, 'The insulin resistance-dysipidemic syndrome: Contribution of visceral obesity and therapeutic implications', *International Journal of Obesity*, 19, Suppl. 1 S76–S86.

9　Munnings, F., 1994, 'Syndrome X: The deadly combination of diseases', *The Physician and Sportsmedicine*, 22(8):63–66.

10　Barnard, R.J., Wen, S.J., 1994, 'Exercise and diet in the prevention and control of the metabolic syndrome', *Sports Medicine*, 18(4): 218–228.

11　Bradley, T.D., 1995, 'Pathophysiological interactions of obesity and sleep apnea', *International Journal of Obesity*, 19(2): 43.

12　Lissner, L. et al., 1991, 'Variability of body weight and health outcomes in the Framingham population', *New England Journal of Medicine*, 324(26): 1839–1844.

13　Brownell, K.D., Wadden, T.A., 1992, 'Etiology and treatment of obesity: understanding a serious, prevalent, and refractory disorder', *Journal of Consulting and Clinical Psychology*, 20(4):505–517.


## 3 Fat physiology

1  Hirsvh, J., Fried, S.K., Edens, N.K., Leibel, R.L., 1989, 'The Fat Cell', *Medical Clinics of North America*, 73(1):83–95.
2  Ailhaud, G., Grimaldi, P., Negrel, R., 1992, 'A molecular view of adipose tissue', *International Journal of Obesity*, 16(Suppl. 2), S17–S21.
3  Raaj, P., et al, 1991, 'Energy costs of lactation and energy balance of well nourished Dutch lactating women: Re-appraisal of the extra energy requirements of lactation', *American Journal of Clinical Nutrition*, 53:612–619.
4  Frisch, R., 1994, 'The right weight: Body fat, menarche and fertility', *Proceedings of the Nutrition Society*, 53:113–129.
5  Swinburn, B., Ravussin, E., 1993, 'Energy balance or fat balance', *American Journal of Clinical Nutrition*, 57(suppl.):766S–71S.
6  Flatt, J-P., 1991, 'Opposite effects of variations in food intake on carbohydrate and fat oxidation in ad libitum fed mice', *Journal of Clinical Biochemistry*, 2:186–192.
7  Wolfe, R.R., Klein, S., Carraro, F., Weber, J-M., 1990, 'Role of triglyceride–fatty acid cycle in controlling fat metabolism in humans during and after exercise', *American Journal of Physiology*, 258: E382-E389.
8  Keim, N.L., Anderson, B.L., Barbieri, T.F., Wu, M-M., 1994, 'Moderate diet restriction alters the substrate and hormone response to exercise', *Medicine and Science in Sports and Exercise*, 26(5): 599–604.


## 4 Bioenergetics and metabolism

1  Ainsworth, B.E., Montoyne, H.J., Leon, A.S., 1994, 'Methods of assessing physical activity during leisure and work', In Bouchard, C., Chephard, R., Stephens, T.(eds) *Physical Activity, Fitness and Health: A Consensus Statement* Human Kinetics, Champaign, Illinois, 46–159.
2  Westerterp, K., Donkers, J.H., Donkers, L.M., Fredrix, W.H.M., Boekhoudt, P., 1995, 'Energy intake, physical activity and body weight: A simulation model', *Brit J Nutr* 73: 337–347.
3  Mole, P.A., 1990, 'Impact of energy intake and exercise on resting metabolic rate', *Sports Medicine*, 10(2):72–87.
4  Thorne, A., 1990, 'Diet induced thermogenesis: An experimental study in healthy and obese individuals', *Acta Chirop Scandinavia*, 558 (Suppl.):56–59.
5  Warwick, P.M., 1989, 'Predicting food energy requirements from estimates of energy expenditure', *Australian Journal of Nutrition and Dietetics*, 46: (Suppl.):S3–S28.

6 Spriet, L.L., 1995, 'Caffeine and performance', *Sports Nutrition*, 5 (Suppl.):S84–99.

7 Bracco, D. et al., 1995, 'Effects of caffeine on energy metabolism, heart rate, and methylxanthine metabolism in lean and obese women', *American Journal of Physiology*, 32:E671–E678.

8 Colquhoun, E. et al., 1993, 'Possible pharmacological approaches to the management of obesity', *Paper presented to the 3rd Annual Meeting of the Australian Society for the Study of Obesity*, Melbourne.

9 Ravussin, E., and Swinburn, B.A., 1993, 'Energy metabolism', In Stunkard A.J., and Wadden, T.A. *Obesity Theory and Therapy*, Raven Press Ltd, NY.

10 Wilmore, J.H., and Costill, D.L., 1994, *Physiology of Sport and Exercise*. Human Kinetics, Champaign, Illinois.

## 5 The role of fat in energy balance

1 Ravussin, E., and Swinburn, B.A. 'Energy metabolism', In Stunkard, A.J., and Wadden, T.A., 1993, *Obesity Theory and Therapy*, Raven Press Ltd, NY.

2 Westerterp, K., Donkers, J.H., Donkers, L.M., Fredrix, W.H.M., Boekhoudt, P., 1995, 'Energy intake, physical activity and body weight: A simulation model', *Brit J Nutr* 73:337–347.

3 Acheson, K.J., Schutz, Y., Bessard, T., Anantharaman, K., Flatt, J-P., 1988, 'Glycogen storage capacity and de novo lipogenesis during massive carbohydrate overfeeding in man', *Am J Clin Nutr* 48:240–247.

4 Westrate, J.A., 1996, 'Fat and obesity', *BNF Nutrition Bulletin*, 21:18–25.

5 Horton, T.J., Drougas, H., Brachey, A. et al., 1995, 'Fat and carbohydrate overfeeding in humans: Different effects on energy storage', *Am J Clin Nutr* 62:19–29.

6 Hellerstedt, W.L., Jeffery, R.W., Murray, D.M., 1990, 'The association between alcohol intake and adiposity in the general population', *American Journal of Epidemiology*, 132:594–611.

7 Stock, M., 1996, 'Alcohol, body weight and energy balance', *BNF Nutrition Bulletin*, 21:49–53.

8 Lieber, C., 1991, 'Perspectives: do alcohol calories count?', *American Journal of Clinical Nutrition*, 54:49–55.

9 Flatt, J-P., Ravussin, E., Acheson, K.J., Jequier, E., 1985, 'Effects of dietary fat on post-prandial substrate oxidation and on carbohydrate and fat balance', *J Clin Invest* 76:1019–1024.

## 6 Measurement and assessment of fatness

1 Hopp, K.D. et al., 1994, 'Is ideal body weight still a clinically relevant concept?', *Medicographica*, 16(3):33–38.

2 Lohman, T.G., 1992, *Advances in body composition assessment*, Human Kinetics, Champaign, Illinois.
3 Jackson, A.S. and Pollock, M.L., 1985, 'Practical assessment of body composition', *The Physician and Sportsmedicine*, 13:77–90.
4 Durnin, J.V. and Womersley, J., 1974, 'Body fat assessment from total body density and its estimation from skinfold thickness: Measurements on 481 men and women aged 16 to 72 years', *British Journal of Nutrition*, 32:77–97.
5 Lohman, T.G., Roche, A.F., Martorell, R., 1988, *Anthropometric standardization reference manual*, Human Kinetics, Champaign, Illinois.
6 Egger, G., 1992, 'The case for using waist-to-hip ratios in standard medical consultations', *Medical Journal of Australia*, 156: 280–5.
7 Lemieux, S. et al., 1995, 'A single threshold value of waist girth to identify non-obese and obese subjects with excess visceral tissue', *International Journal of Obesity*, 19(2):29.
8 McLean, M.E.J., Han, T.S., Morrison, C.E., 1995, 'Waist circumference as a measure for indicating need for weight management', *British Medical Journal*, 31:1158–161.
9 Valdez, R., Seidell, J.C., Ahn, Y.I., and Weiss, K.M., 1993, 'A new index of abdominal adiposity as an indicator of risk for cardiovascular disease: A cross population study', *International Journal of Obesity*, 17:77–82.
10 Kahn, H.S., 1993, 'Choosing an index for abdominal obesity: An opportunity for epidemiological clarification', *Journal of Clinical Epidemiology*, 46:491–494.

## 7 Influences on overfatness and obesity

1 Hawks, S.R., Richins, P., 1994, 'Toward a new paradigm for the management of obesity', *Journal of Health Education*, 25(3):147–153.
2 Flatt, J-P., 1995, 'Body composition, respiratory quotient, and weight maintenance', *American Journal of Clinical Nutrition*, 62(Suppl.):1107S–1117S.
3 Alpert, S., 1990, 'Growth, thermogenesis, and hyperphagia', *American Journal of Clinical Nutrition*, 52:784–792.
4 Swinburn, B., Ravussin, E., 1993, 'Energy metabolism', In Stunkard, A.J. and Wadden, T.A. *Obesity: Theory and Therapy* (2nd Edition), Raven Press, NY.
5 Flatt, J-P., 1988, 'Importance of nutrient balance in body weight regulation', *Diabetes and Metabolism Reviews*, 6:571–81.
6 Blair, S.N., 1994, 'Physical activity, physical fitness and health', *Research Quarterly in Exercise and Sport*, 64(4): 365–376.
7 Prentice, A.M., Goldberg, G.R., Jebb, S.A., Black, A.E., Murgatroyd, P.R., 1991, 'Physiological responses to slimming', *Proceedings of the Nutrition Society*, 50:441–458.
8 Bouchard, C., 1993, 'The etiology of obesity: Genetic and non genetic factors', *American Journal of Clinical Nutrition*, 60: 171–81.

9 Rebuffe-Scrive, M., Enk, L., Crona, N. et al., 1985, 'Fat cell metabolism in different regions in women: Effect of menstrual cycle, pregnancy and lactation', *Journal of Clinical Investigation*, 75:1973–1976.

10 Tuten, C., Petosa, R., Sargent, R., Weston, A., 1995, 'Biracial differences in physical activity and body composition', *Obesity Research*, 3(4):313–318.

11 Brownell, K.D., Wadden, T.A., 1992, 'Etiology and treatment of obesity: Understanding a serious, prevalent, and refractory disorder', *Journal of Consulting and Clinical Psychology*, 60: 505–517.

## 8 Dietary fat and how to reduce it

1 Australian Nutrition Foundation, 1995, *The Healthy Eating Pyramid*, Sydney.

2 National Health and Medical Research Council, 1992, *Dietary Guidelines for Australians*, Australian Government Publishing Service, Canberra.

3 Stanton, R., 1994, *Eating for Peak Performance* (2nd edn), Allen & Unwin, Sydney.

4 Hill, J.O., 1995, 'Nutrient intake and metabolism', *Obesity Research*, 3:314S.

5 Swinburn, B. and Ravussin, E., 1993, 'Energy balance or fat balance', *American Journal of Clinical Nutrition*, 57(Suppl.):766S–771S.

6 National Health and Medical Research Council, 1991, *Report on the role of polyunsaturated fats in the Australian diet*, Australian Government Publishing Service, Canberra.

7 Egger, G. and Stanton, R., 1992, *The GutBuster Waist Loss Guide*, Allen & Unwin, Sydney.

8 Baghurst, K.I., Record, S.J. and Baghurst, P.A. et al., 1993, 'What are Australians eating?' *Results of the 1985 & 1990 Victorian nutrition surveys*, Food and Nutrition Program, Victoria.

9 Pan, D.A., Hulbert, A.J. and Storlien, L.H., 1994, 'Dietary fats, membrane phospholipids and obesity', *Journal of Nutrition*, 124:1555–1565.

10 National Heart Foundation of Australia, 1994, *Dietary fatty acids and blood cholesterol*, NHF, Canberra.

11 Errasmus, U., 1986, *Fats and oils*, Alive Books, Vancouver.

12 Katan, M.B., 1995, 'Fish and heart disease', *New England Journal of Medicine*, 332(15): 1024–1025.

13 Somerset, S., 1994, 'Trans-fatty acid consumption in Australia', *Food Australia*, 46(12):564–566.

14 Baghurst, K., 1995, 'Getting it right: Just what advice should we give about fat reduction?' *Perspectives in Food and Nutrition*, 1:12–15.

15 Dobson, A.J., Blijlevens, R., Alexander, H.M. et al., 1993, 'Short fat questionnaire: A self administered measure of fat intake', *Australian Journal of Public Health*, 17:144–149.

16 Stanton, R., 1994, *Fat & Fibre Counter*, Wilkinson Books, Sydney.

17 'Food label claims: what do they mean?' February, 1994, *Choice*.

18 National Food Authority, 1994, *Code of Practice on nutrient claims in food labels and in advertisements*, Canberra.
19 Kristal, A.R. et al., 1990, 'Patterns of dietary behavior associated with selecting diets low in fat: Reliability and validity of a behavioral approach to dietary assessment', *Journal of the American Dietetic Association*, 90:214–220.
20 Swinburn, B., 1995, *Fat Countdown*, University of Auckland, School of Community Health.
21 Kristal, A.R. et al., 1992, 'Long-term maintenance of a low-fat diet: Durability of fat related dietary habits in the Women's Health Trial', *Journal of the American Dietetic Association*, 92:553–559.
22 Mela, D.J., 1993, 'Consumer estimates of the energy from fat in common foods', *European Journal of Clinical Nutrition*, 47:735–740.
23 Shide, D.J. and Rolls, B.J., 1995, 'Information about the fat content of preloads influences energy intake in healthy women', *Journal of the American Dietetic Association*, 95:993–8.

## 9 Dietary carbohydrate and how to increase it

1 Southgate, D., June, 1995, 'The elusive definition of carbohydrates', *Proceedings of Carbohydrates and Health Symposium*, International Life Sciences Institute, Sydney.
2 Stephen, A.M. et al., 1995, 'Intake of carbohydrate and its components—international comparisons, trends over time and effects of changing to low-fat diets', *American Journal of Clinical Nutrition*, 62:851S–67S.
3 Topping, D., Wong, S.H., 1994, 'Preventative and therapeutic aspects of dietary fibre', In Vobecky, J., and Wahlqvist, M. (eds), *Medical Practice of Preventative Nutrition*, Smith and Gordon, London.
4 Stanton, R., Bolin, T., 1994, *Windbreaks*, Wilkinson Books, Sydney.
5 Englyst, H.N., and Kingman, S.M., 1992, 'Classification and measurement of nutritionally important starch fractions', *European Journal of Clinical Nutrition*, 26:S33–S50.
6 Macdonald, N., 6 June, 1995, 'Glycaemic index—an update and overview', *Nutrition issues and Abstracts*.
7 Foster-Powell, K., Brand Miller, J., 1995, 'International tables of glycaemic index', *American Journal of Clinical Nutrition*, 62:871S–93S.
8 Wolver, T. et al., 1991, 'The glycaemic index: Methodology and clinical implications', *American Journal of Clinical Nutrition*, 54:846–54.
9 Holt, S., Brand Miller, J., 1995, 'Increased insulin responses to ingested foods are associated with lessened satiety', *Appetite*, 24:43–54.
10 Brand Miller, J., Forster-Powell, K. and Colaguri, S., 1996, *The GI Factor*, Hodder & Stoughton, Sydney.
11 Higginson, J., Oettle, A.G., 1960, 'Cancer incidence in Bantu and 'Cape Coloured' races in South Africa: Report of a cancer survey in the Transvaal (1953–1955)', *Journal of the National Cancer Institute*, 24:589–671.

12  Hill, J., Prentice, A., 1995, 'Sugar and body weight regulation', *American Journal of Clinical Nutrition*, 62(Suppl.):264S–274S.

## 10  Hunger, appetite and eating behaviour

1  Blundell, J., Hill, A., 1992, 'Dexfenfluramine and appetite in humans', *International Journal of Obesity*, 16(Suppl.3):S51-S59.
2  Brand Miller, J., 1994, *Nutrition Issues & Abstracts*, 1 March.
3  Hoebel, B., Hernandez, L., 1993, 'Basic neural mechanisms of feeding and weight regulation', In Stunkard, A., and Wadden, T.A. (eds) *Obesity: Theory and Therapy*, (2nd edn), Raven Press, New York, p. 45.
4  Bray, G., 1994, 'Appetite control in humans', In Fernstrom, J. & Miller, G. (eds) *Appetite and body weight regulation*, ILSI Publications, NY.
5  Sclafani, A., 1993, 'Dietary Obesity', In Stunkard, A. & Wadden, T. (eds) *Obesity: Theory and Therapy*, (2nd edn) Raven Press, New York, p. 133.
6  Pollock, N.J., 1995, 'Social fattening patterns in the Pacific: The positive side of obesity—A Nauru case study', In de Garine, I. and Pollock, N.J. (eds), *Social Aspects of Obesity*, Gordon and Breach, London.
7  Greeno, C., Wing, R., 1994, 'Stress-Induced Eating', *Psychological Bulletin*. 115(3):444–464.
8  Blundell, J.E., Hill, A.J., Rogers, P.J., 1988, 'Hunger and the satiety cascade—their importance to food acceptance in the late 20th century', In Thompson, D. (ed.) *Food Acceptability*, Elsevier, Amsterdam, pp. 223–250.
9  Green, S.M., Blundell, J.E., 1995, 'Comparison of the perceived fillingness and actual intake of snack foods', *International Journal of Obesity*, 19(2):28.
10  O'Dea, K., 1992, 'Obesity and diabetes in "the land of milk and honey" ', *Diabetes/Metabolism Reviews*, 8(4):373–388.
11  Blundell, J.E. et al., 1993, 'Dietary fat and the control of energy intake: Evaluating the effects of fat on meal size and postmeal satiety', *American Journal of Clinical Nutrition*, 57(suppl.):772S–778S.
12  Wurtman, J.J., 1984, 'The involvement of brain seratonin in excessive carbohydrate snacking by obese carbohydrate cravers', *Journal of the American Dietetic Association*, 84:1004–7.
13  Drewnowski, A., et al., 1992, 'Food preferences in human obesity: carbohydrates versus fats', *Appetite*, 18:207–21.
14  Burley, V. et al., 1994, 'Patterns of appetite control following high fibre breakfast: Comparison of soluble and insoluble fibre', *International Journal of Obesity*, 18(2 Suppl.):134.
15  Turconi, G. et al., 1993, 'High-calorie fibre-rich breakfast: Its effect on satiety', *Journal of Human Nutrition & Dietetics* 6:245–252.
16  Hill, A.J. and Blundell, J.E., 1986, 'Macronutrients and satiety: effects

of a high-protein or high-carbohydrate meal on subjective motivation to eat', *Nutrition Behaviour*, 3:133–44.

17 de Castro, J.M., Orozco, S., 1990, 'Moderate alcohol intake and spontaneous eating patterns of humans: Evidence of unregulated supplementation', *American Journal of Clinical Nutrition*, 52:246–253.

18 Chen, L.N.A. and Parham, E.S., 1991, 'College students use of high-intensity sweeteners is not consistently associated with sugar consumption', *Journal of the American Dietetic Association*, 91:686–90.

19 Drewnowski, A., 1995, 'Intense sweeteners and the control of appetite', *Nutrition Reviews*, 53(1):1–7.

20 Poppit, S.D. and Prentice, A.M., 1996 'Energy density and its role in the control of food intake: Evidence from metabolic and community studies', *Appetite*, 26:153–74.

21 Rolls, B., 1994, 'Role of fat substitutes in obesity prevention and treatment', *International Journal of Obesity*, 18(2 Suppl.):42.

22 Westrate, J. and van het Hof, K.H., 1995, 'Sucrose polyester and plasma carotenoid concentrations in healthy subjects', *American Journal of Clinical Nutrition*, 62(3):591–7.

23 Drewnowski, A., 1995, 'Energy intake and sensory properties of food', *American Journal of Clinical Nutrition*, 62(suppl.):1081S–1085S.

24 Holt, S.H.A. et al., 1995, 'A satiety index of common foods', *European Journal of Clinical Nutrition*, 49:675–690.

## 11 Fad diets and dieting for fat loss

1 Swinburn, B., 1995, 'Fats', *Nutrition Notes and Reviews*.
2 Berland, T., 1986, *Rating the Diets*, Signet Books, New York.
3 Stanton, R., 1991, *The Diet Dilemma*, Allen & Unwin, Sydney.
4 *National Council Against Food Fraud, Newsletter*, March/April 1987.

## 12 Physical activity and fat loss

1 Pacy, P.J., Webster, J., Garrow, J.S., 1986, 'Exercise and obesity', *Sports Medicine*. 3: 89–113.
2 Andrews, J.F., 1991, 'Exercise for slimming', *Proceedings of the Nutrition Society*, 50:459–471.
3 Stephanick, M.L., 1993, 'Exercise and Weight Control', *Exercise and Sports Science Review*, 21:363–396.
4 Bouchard, C., 1995, 'Individual differences in the response to regular exercise', *International Journal of Obesity*, 19(Suppl. 4):S5–8.
5 Wilmore, J.H., Costill, D.L., 1994, *Physiology of sport and exercise*, Human Kinetics, Illinois.
6 Coleman, E., 1995, 'Fat burning and exercise', *Sports Medicine Digest*, March: 7.
7 Glasser, G.A., 1995, 'Burning carbohydrate to lose fat', *Sports Medicine Digest*, March: 7.

8   Tremblay, A., Simoneau, J.A., Bouchard, C., 1994, 'Impact of exercise intensity on body fatness and skeletal muscle metabolism', *Metabolism*, 43(7):814–818.

9   Romijn, J.A. et al., 1993, 'Regulation of endogenous fat and carbohydrate metabolism in relation to exercise intensity and duration', *American Journal of Physiology*, 265: E380–E341.

10  Kelly, D., 1995, 'The regulation of glucose uptake and oxidation during exercise', *International Journal of Obesity*, 19(Suppl. 4):S5–8.

11  Turcotte, L.P., Richter, E.A., Kiens, B., 1992, 'Increased plasma FFA uptake and oxidation during prolonged exercise in trained vs. untrained humans', *American Journal of Physiology*, E791–E799.

12  Hurley, B.F. et al., 1986, 'Muscle triglyceride utilisation during exercise: Effect of training', *Journal of Applied Physiology*, 60 (2):562–567.

13  Martin, J.M. et al., 1993, 'Effect of endurance training on plasma free fatty acid turnover and oxidation during exercise', *American Journal of Physiology*, 265:E708–E714.

14  Kiens, B. et al., 1993, 'Skeletal muscle utilisation during sub maximal exercise in man: Effect of endurance training', *Journal of Physiology*, 469:459–478.

15  Wolfe, R.R. et al., 1990, 'Role of triglyceride-fatty acid cycle in controlling fat metabolism in humans during and after exercise', *American Journal of Physiology*, 258:E382–E389.

16  Blair, S., 1994, 'Physical activity, physical fitness and health', *Research Quarterly in Exercise and Sport*, 64(4):365–376.

17  Jakicic, J.M., Wing, R.R., Butler, B.A., Robertson, R.J., 1995, 'Prescribing exercise in multiple short bouts versus one continuous bout: effects on adherence, cardiorespiratory fitness, and weight loss in overweight men', *International Journal of Obesity*, 19: 893–901.

## 13  Individualised movement prescription for fat loss

1   Bouchard, C., 1995, 'Individual differences in the response to regular exercise', *International Journal of Obesity*, 19(4):S5–S9.

2   Bourdin, M. et al., 1993, 'Influence of training, sex, age and body mass on the energy cost of running', *European Journal of Applied Physiology*, 66:439–444.

3   Egger, G., 1994, 'Heterogeneity of the fat loss response to exercise', *Australian Society for the Study of Obesity*, Annual Conference, Brisbane.

4   Tarnopolsky, M.A., Atkinson, S.A., Phillips, S.M., and McDougall, J.D., 1995, 'Carbohydrate loading and metabolism during exercise in men and women', *Journal of Applied Physiology*, 78(4):1360–1368.

5   Tremblay, A., Despres, J-P., LeBlanc, C., Bouchard, C., 1984, 'Sex dimorphism in fat loss in response to exercise training', *Journal of Obesity and Weight Regulation*, 3:193–203.

6   King, N., Blundell, J.E., 1995, 'Individual differences in substrate

oxidation and macronutrient selection: Correlation between RQ and FQ', *International Journal of Obesity*, 19(2): 33.

7　Gleim, G.W., 1993, 'Exercise is not an effective weight loss modality in women', *Journal of the American College of Nutrition*, 12(4): 363–367.

8　Blair, S., 1994, 'Physical activity, physical fitness and health', *Research Quarterly in Exercise and Sport*, 64(4):365–376.

9　Shephard, R.J., 1992, 'Fat metabolism, exercise and the cold', *Canadian Journal of Sports Science*, 17(2):83–90.

10　Keim, N.L. et al., 1992, 'Moderate diet restriction alters substrate and hormone response to exercise', *Medicine and Science in Sports and Exercise*, 26(5); 599–604.

11　Lightman, S.W. et al., 1992, 'Discrepancy between self-reported and actual caloric intake and exercise in obese subjects', *New England Journal of Medicine*, 27:1893–1898.

12　Dausch, J.D., 1992, 'The problem of obesity: Fundamental concepts of energy metabolism gone awry', *Critical Reviews in Food Science and Nutrition*, 31(4):271–298.

13　Raben, A. et al., 1994, 'Evidence for an abnormal postprandial response to a high fat meal in women predisposed to obesity', *American Journal of Physiology*, 267: E549–E559.

14　Kiens, B. et al., 1993, 'Skeletal muscle utilisation during sub maximal exercise in man: Effect of endurance training', *Journal of Physiology*, 469:459–478.

15　Treuth, M.S. et al., 1994, 'Effects of strength training on total and regional body composition in older men', *Journal of Applied Physiology*, 77(2):614–620.

16　Egger, G. and Champion, N., 1990, *The Fitness Leader's Handbook* (2nd Edition), Kangaroo Press, Sydney.

17　Walberg, J.L., 1989, 'Aerobic exercise and resistance weight-training during weight reduction', *Sports Medicine*, 47:343–356.

## 14　Physiological adjustment and maintenance of fat loss

1　Keys, A. et al, 1950, *The Biology of Human Starvation, Vol 1*. University of Minnesota Press: Minneapolis.

2　Merkt, J.R., Taylor, C.R., 1994, ' "Metabolic switch" for desert survival', *Proceedings of the National Academy of Science USA*, 91:12313–12316.

3　Leibel, R.L., Rosenbaum, M., Hirsch, J., 1995, 'Changes in energy expenditure resulting from altered body weight', *New England Journal of Medicine*, 332:621–8.

4　Prentice, A.M. et al., 1991, 'Physiological responses to slimming', *Proceedings of the Nutrition Society*, 50:441–458.

5　Garrow, J., 1995, 'Exercise in the treatment of obesity: A marginal contribution', *International Journal of Obesity*, 19(Suppl. 4):S126–S130.

6　Ballor, D.L., and Poehlman, E.T., 1994, 'Exercise training enhances fat-free mass preservation during diet-induced weight loss: A meta-analytical finding', *International Journal of Obesity and Related Metabolic Disorders,* 18(1):35–40.

7 Garrow, J.S., Summerbell, C.D., 1995, 'Meta-analysis: effects of exercise, with or without dieting, on the body composition of overweight subjects', *European Journal of Clinical Nutrition,* 49:1–10.

8 Cannon, G., Einzig, H., 1983, *Dieting Makes You Fat,* Century Publishing, London.

## 15 Environmental influences

1 Hodge, A.M. et al., 1995, 'Modernity and obesity in coastal and highland Papua New Guinea', *International Journal of Obesity,* 19:154–161.

2 Chapman, S., 1995, 'Unwrapping gossamer with boxing gloves', *British Medical Journal,* 311:989.

3 Watson, M.J. et al., 1992, 'Fat content of untrimmed beef and lamb cuts 2: Influence of outlet and neighbourhood over a year', *Food Australia,* 44:516–518.

4 NHF 'Pick the Tick' Program, 1995, *Heart Health,* National Heart Foundation.

5 BIS Schrapnel Report, 1994, *Fast Food in Australia,* Sydney.

6 Alexander, H.M. et al., 1995, *Hunter region heart disease prevention programme: Risk factor prevalence study,* 1994 Data Book, University of Newcastle, NSW.

7 Aastrand, P-O., 1994, 'Physical activity and fitness: Evolutionary perspective and trends for the future', In Bouchard, C., Shephard, R., and Stephens, T. (eds) *Physical Activity, Fitness and Health: International Proceedings and Consensus Statement,* Human Kinetics, Champaigne Illinois.

8 Dwyer, T., Coonan, W., 1985, 'The daily PE program', *ACHPER Report,* Adelaide.

9 Egger, G., 'Men's health in the middle years', In Galbally, R. (ed.) *Health Promotion: refocusing the issue,* Macmillan Melbourne (in press).

10 Saris, W., September, 1995, 'Exercise and obesity', *Paper presented to the Australian Society for the Study of Obesity,* Annual Conference, Melbourne.

11 Parish, A.M., 1995, 'Evaluation of a correspondence fat loss program for men', Unpublished Master's Thesis, University of Wollongong, School of Health and Medical Sciences.

12 Egger, G., Stanton, R., 1995, *GutBuster 2: The High Energy Guide,* Allen & Unwin, Sydney.

13 Epstein, L.H. et al., 1995, 'Effects of decreasing sedentary behavior and increasing activity on weight change in obese children', *Health Psychology,* 14(2):109–115.

14 Egger, G., 1995, *The attitude of middle-aged men to exercise,* Report for VICFIT, Department of Recreation and Sport, Melbourne.

## 16 Biological influences

1 Bouchard, C., 1991, 'Heredity and the path to overweight and obesity', *Medicine and Science in Sports and Exercise*, 23(3):285–291.
2 Falciglia, G.A., Norton, P.A., 1994, 'Evidence for a genetic influence on preference for some foods', *Journal of the American Dietetic Association*, 94(2):154–158.
3 Coleman, D.L., 1973, 'Obesity and diabetes: Two mutant genes causing diabetes–obesity syndromes in mice', *Diabetologia*, 9:294–298.
4 Zhang, Y. et al., 1995, 'Positional cloning of the mouse obese gene and its human analogue', *Nature*, 372, 1st December, 1994.
5 Halaas, J.L. et al., 1995, 'Weight reducing effects of the plasma protein encoded by the obese gene', *Science*, 269:543–546.
6 Rebuffe-Scrive, M., Andersson, B., Olbe, L., Bjorntorp, P., 1989, 'Metabolism of adipose tissue in intra-abdominal depots of non obese men and women', *Metabolism*, 38:453–458.
7 Rossner, S., Ohlin, A., 1995, 'Pregnancy as a risk factor for obesity: Lessons from the Stockholm and weight development study', *Obesity Research*, 3:276S–278S.
8 Gleim, G.W., 1993, 'Exercise is not an effective weight loss modality in women', *Journal of the American College of Nutrition*, 12(4):363–367.
9 Klein, A.M., 1994, *Little Big Men*, University of NY Press, NY.
10 Treuth, M.S. et al., 1994, 'Effects of strength training on total and regional body composition in older men', *Journal of Applied Physiology*, 77(2): 614–620.
11 Roberts, S.B. et al., 1994, 'Control of food intake in older men', *Journal of the American Medical Association*, 272:1601–1606.

## 17 Behavioural influences

1 Hirsch, J., 1975, 'The psychological consequences of obesity', In Bray G.A. (ed.) *Obesity in Perspective: A Conference*, US Govt Printing Office.
2 Streigel-Moore, R., Rodin, J., 1986, 'The influence of psychological variables in obesity', In Brownell, K.D. and Foreyt, J.P. (eds), *Handbook of Eating Disorders*, Basic Books, NY.
3 Gurin, J., 1989, 'Leaner, not lighter—Why you need to rethink your beliefs about dieting before you start', *Psychology Today*, June.
4 Bray, G.A., 'Effects of obesity on health and happiness', In Brownell, K.D. and Foreyt, J.P. (eds), *Handbook of Eating Disorders*, Basic Books, NY.
5 Tupling, H., 1991, *A weight off your mind*, Bantam, Sydney.
6 Stuart, R.B., 1980, 'Weight loss and beyond: Are they taking it off and keeping it off?', In Parks, O., Davidson, L. and Davidson, S.M. (eds), *Behavioural Medicine: Changing Health Lifestyles*, Mazel, NY.

7 Brownell, K.D. and Foreyt, J.P. (eds), 1986, *Handbook of Eating Disorders*, Basic Books, NY.

8 Ellis, A., Harper, R.A., 1975, *A new guide to rational living*, Wilshire Books, LA.

9 Seligman, M., 1991, *Learned Optimism*, Random House, NY.

10 Seligman, M., 1975, *Learned Helplessness*, Freeman, San Francisco.

11 Rogers, P.J., Green, M.W., 1993, 'Dieting, dietary restraint and cognitive performance', *British Journal of Clinical Psychology*, 32: 113–116.

12 Biener, L., Heaton, A., 1995, 'Women dieters of normal weight: Their motives, goals, and risks', *American Journal of Public Health*, 85: 714–717.

13 Orbach, S., 1978, *Fat is a Feminist Issue*, Hamlyn, NY.

14 Wolfe, N., 1990, *The Beauty Myth*, Chatto & Windus, NY.

15 Wysoker, E., 1994, 'Women's experience losing weight and gaining the lost weight back', *International Journal of Obesity*, 18(2):80.

## 18 Critical periods for fat gain and relapse

1 LeBow, M.D., 1991, *Overweight children: Helping your child achieve lifetime weight control*, Insight Books, NY.

2 Dietz, W., 1996, 'The fattening effects of television', *Waist Watch*, 13:1.

3 Epstein, L. et al., 1995, 'Effects of decreasing sedentary behaviour and increasing activity on weight change in obese children', *Health Psychology*, 14(2):109–115.

4 Raaj, P. et al., 1991, 'Energy costs of lactation and energy balance of well nourished Dutch lactating women: Re-appraisal of the energy requirements of lactation', *American Journal of Clinical Nutrition*, 53:612–619.

5 Berg, J., 1995, 'Bigger babies—a public health blunder?', *Healthy Weight Journal*, 9(5):84.

6 Frisch, R., 1994, 'The right body weight: body fat, menarche and fertility', *Proceedings of the Nutrition Society*, 53:113–129.

7 Sherriff, J.L. and Hartmann, P.E., 1995, 'Energy expenditure during lactation—a review of the literature', *Australian Journal of Nutrition and Dietetics*, 52(4):187–200.

8 Rossner, S. and Ohlin, A., 1995, 'Pregnancy as a risk factor for obesity: Lessons from the Stockholm Pregnancy and Weight Development Study', *Obesity Research*, 3(Suppl. 2):267S–276S.

9 Cooney, S., 1992, *The menopause industry: A guide to medicine's 'discovery' of the mid-life woman*, Prentice Hall, NY.

10 Treuth, M.S. et al., 1995, 'Energy expenditure and substrate utilisation in older women after strength training: 24h calorimeter result', *Journal of Applied Physiology*, 78(6):2140–2146.

11 Greeno, G. and Wing, R.R., 1994, 'Stress induced eating', *Psychological Bulletin*, 115(3):444–464.

12  Van Strien, T. et al., 1986, 'Life events, emotional eating and change in body mass index', *International Journal of Obesity*, 10:29–35.

13  NHANES, 1992, *International Journal of Obesity*, 16:745–753.

14  Truswell, S., 1987, *Marriage and overweight*, Sydney University Report.

15  Raushenbach, B., Sobal, J., Frongillo, E.A. Jr., 1995, 'The influence of change in marital status on weight change over 1 year', *Obesity Research*, 3(4): 319–328.

16  Swan, G.E., Carmelli, D., 1995, 'Characteristics associated with excessive weight gain after smoking cessation in men', *American Journal of Public Health*, 85(1):73–77.

17  Egger, G. and Stanton, R., 1993, *The GutBuster 'Waist Loss' Guide for Men*, Allen & Unwin, Sydney.

18  Egger, G. and Stanton, R., 1995, *GutBuster 2: The high energy guide*, Allen & Unwin, Sydney.

19  Westerterp-Plantenga, M.S., Van Den Heuvel, E., Wouters, L., Ten Door, F.T., 1992, 'Diet-induced thermogenesis and cumulative food intake curves as a function of familiarity with food and dietary restraint in humans', *Physiology and Behavior*, 51:457–465.

20  Australian Medical Association, 1994, *Guide to Medicines and Drugs*, Sydney.

21  Kirschenbaum, D.S., Fitzgibbon, M.L., 1995, 'Controversy about the treatment of obesity: Criticisms and challenges?', *Behavior Therapy*, 26:43–68.

22  Kayman, S., Bruvoid, W., and Stern, J.S., 1990, 'Maintenance and relapse after weight loss in women: Behavioral aspects', *American Journal of Clinical Nutrition*, 52:800–807.

23  Greeno, G. and Wing, R.R., 1994, 'Stress induced eating', *Psychological Bulletin*, 115(3):444–464.

24  Wadden, T., 1994, 'Obesity prevention following the treatment of obesity: Behavioral and psychological factors', *Paper presented to the 7th International Conference on Obesity*, Toronto, Canada.

## 19  Drugs and surgical treatment

1  American Medical Association, 1990, 'Drugs used in obesity', *Drug Evaluations Subscriptions*, 3(6):1–616.

2  Kraal, J.G., 1989, 'Surgical treatment of obesity', *Medical Clinics of North America*, 73(1):251–264.

3  Ravussin, E. and Bogardus, C., 1989, 'Essential obesity and the pathogenic role of a low metabolic rate', In *Nutrition and the Origins of Disease*, Academic Press, NY, pp.145–160.

4  Silverstone, T., 1993, 'The place of appetite suppressant drugs in the treatment of obesity', In Stunkard, A.J. and Wadden, T.A. (eds) *Obesity: Theory and Therapy*, Raven Press Ltd, NY.

5  Bjorntorp, P., 1992, 'Treatment of obesity', *International Journal of Obesity*, 16(Suppl.3):S81–84.

6   Fobi, M., 1993, 'Operations that are questionable for control of obesity', *Obesity Surgery*, 3:2.

## 20 Eating disorders

1   Brownell, K.D. and Foreyt, J.P. (eds), 1986, *Handbook of eating disorders*, Basic Books, NY.
2   e.g. *International Journal of Eating Disorders*.
3   Fussel, S., 1989, *Muscle*, Pan Books, NY.
4   Klein, A.M., 1993, *Little Big Men: Bodybuilding subculture and gender construction*, State University of New York Press, NY.
5   Strober, M., 1986, 'Anorexia Nervosa: History and psychological concepts', In Brownell, K.D. and Foreyt, J.P. (eds), *Handbook of eating disorders*, Basic Books, NY.
6   Horm, J., Anderson, K., 1993, 'Who in America is trying to lose weight?', *Annals of Internal Medicine*, 119:672–676.
7   *Diagnostic and Standards Manual of Mental Disorders*, 4th Edition, 1994, American Psychiatric Association.
8   Boskin-White, M., White, W.C., 1986, 'Bulimarexia: A historical-socio-cultural perspective', In Brownell, K.D. and Foreyt, J.P. (eds), *Handbook of eating disorders*, Basic Books, NY.
9   Wooley, S.C., and Kearney-Cooke, A., 1986, 'Intensive treatment of bulimia and body-image disturbance', In Brownell, K.D. and Foreyt, J.P. (eds), *Handbook of eating disorders*, Basic Books, NY.
10  Hermann, J.L., 1995, *Seminar on psychotherapy for adult survivors of sexual abuse*, Sydney.
11  Goodron, G.K. and Foreyt, J.P., 1991, 'Why treatments for obesity don't last', *Journal of the American Dietetic Association*, 91(10).

## 21 Ethical issues in obesity treatment

1   Garner, D.M. and Wooley, S.C., 1991, 'Confronting the failure of behavioural and dietary treatments for obesity', *Clinical Psychology Review*, 11 (6):729–80.
2   Wooley, S.C. and Wooley, O.W., 1983, 'Should obesity be treated at all?' *Psychiatric Annals*, 13(11):884–5, 888; Lustig, A., 1991, 'Weight loss programs: Failing to meet ethical standards?', *Journal of the American Dietetic Association*, 91(10): 1252–4.
3   Wooley, S.C., Wooley, O.W. and Dyrenforth, S.R., 1979, 'Theoretical, practical and social issues in behavioural treatments of obesity', *Journal of Applied Behaviour Analysis*, 12:3–25.
4   Lustig, A., 1991, 'Weight loss programs: Failing to meet ethical standards?', *Journal of the American Dietetic Association*, 91(10): 1252–4.
5   Begley, C.E., 1991, 'Government should strengthen regulation in the

weight loss industry', *Journal of the American Dietetic Association*, 91:255–7.

6  Wooley, S.C. and Garner, D.M., 1991, 'Obesity treatment: The high cost of false hope', *Journal of the American Dietetic Association*, 91:1248–51.

7  Wooley, S.C. and Wooley, O.W., 1983, 'Should obesity be treated at all?' *Psychiatric Annals*, 13(11):884–5, 888.

# Index